"With *The Kissing Bug*, Daisy Hernández takes her place alongside great science writers like Rebecca Skloot and Mary Roach, immersing herself in the deeply personal subject of a deadly insect-borne disease that haunted her own family. It's a tender and compelling personal saga, an incisive work of investigative journalism, and an absolutely essential perspective on global migration, poverty, and pandemics."

—AMY STEWART, author of *Wicked Bugs*

"The question *The Kissing Bug* investigates is timely: Who does the United States take care of, and who does it leave behind? Through the personal story of Hernández's family and countless interviews that include patients and epidemiologists, the inequity of the healthcare system is exposed. Hernández writes to the heart of the story with immense tenderness, compassion, and intelligence. A riveting read."

—ANGIE CRUZ, author of *Dominicana*

"Daisy Hernández introduces us to the most important bug you've probably never heard of. Authoritative and gripping at the same time, *The Kissing Bug* is a deft mix of family archaeology, parasite detective story, and American reckoning. A much-needed addition to the canon."

—DANIELLE OFRI, MD, PhD, author of *When We Do Harm: A Doctor Confronts Medical Error*

"In this wonderful story, Daisy Hernández describes how the bite of a kissing bug impacted the life of her beloved auntie and mentor. She dives into the fascinating history of the kissing bug disease and how it destroys the lives of the bitten, often poor immigrants who fall through the cracks of our for-profit medical industry. An engaging, eye-opening read for anyone looking to learn more about the human suffering caused by the collision of a parasite and years of neglect by the United States' medical system."

—KRIS NEWBY, author of *Bitten: The Secret History of Lyme Disease and Biological Weapons*

THE KISSING BUG

Published by Tin House, Portland, Oregon

Distributed by W. W. Norton & Company

Library of Congress Cataloging-in-Publication Data

Names: Hernández, Daisy, author.
Title: The kissing bug : a true story of a family, an insect, and a
    nation's neglect of a deadly disease / Daisy Hernández.
Description: Portland : Tin House, 2021. | Includes bibliographical
    references and index.
Identifiers: LCCN 2020057435 | ISBN 9781951142520 (hardcover) | ISBN
    9781951142537 (ebook)
Subjects: LCSH: Chagas' disease. | Communicable diseases--United
    States--Social aspects. | Communicable diseases--United
    States--Political aspects. | Epidemics--United States--History--20th
    century. | Families--Health and hygiene--Biography.
Classification: LCC RC124.4 .H47 2021 | DDC 616.9/363--dc23
LC record available at https://lccn.loc.gov/2020057435

First US Edition 2021
Printed in the USA
Interior design by Diane Chonette
Cover images: © Nature Picture Library / Alamy; © Rawpixel

www.tinhouse.com

THE
KISSING
BUG

A True Story of a Family, an Insect, and

a Nation's Neglect of a Deadly Disease

DAISY HERNÁNDEZ

 TIN HOUSE / Portland, Oregon

For Maya Durga

Any woman's death diminishes me.

—ADRIENNE RICH

There is a prayer in the act of writing.

—CHERRÍE MORAGA

CONTENTS

IN SEARCH OF OTHER FAMILIES

A WORD SHE WHISPERS

The New York City hospital is a black, cavernous mouth. I am six, and I am not afraid. Bolting from the elevator, I run down the corridor ahead of my mother and baby sister, my sneakers squealing on the clean floors. The doors are half-open. The doors are invitations. A cuarto here belongs to us. The room holds Tía Dora, my mother's sister, my auntie-mother.

A single window in the room stretches toward the ceiling, and Tía Dora is there with her pointy chin and thin face. The Spanish words tiptoe from her mouth. "Mi vida," she murmurs when she sees my mother.

Tía Dora rises onto her elbows. The gown sways on her small frame. She smiles at me with approval. My mother has combed my black hair into two ponytails. My sister, almost a year old, giggles in her summer dress. Outside the Manhattan heat licks our faces, but in the hospital, in my auntie's room, the cold air bites our ears.

The doctors have sewn a line of dark stars across Tía Dora's belly. Las cicatrices. And they have told her a word my mother whispers when she thinks I am not listening: Chagas.

...

No one in the hospital that day, or for many years after, told me that Chagas is a parasitic disease. Transmitted to humans by triatomine insects called kissing bugs, the parasite can often be eradicated with medication when a person is initially infected. Few people, though, are diagnosed and fewer receive treatment, which means the single-celled parasite *Trypanosoma cruzi* can spend up to thirty years in the human body, quietly interrupting the electric currents of the heart, devouring the heart muscle, leaving behind pockets where once healthy tissue existed. In the worst cases, the heart can eventually die.

The illness has come to be known in English as the kissing bug disease.

...

The corazón, the heart, is an accordion. It expands inside the rib cage, then squeezes. It belts out the familiar tune, the sacred thrumming that physicians in the early nineteenth century compared to a whip or, depending on the disease, a dog's tongue lapping. In 1836, Dr. Peter Mere Latham insisted that the musical movements of the heart could not be rendered in paragraphs. "It is useless to describe them," he wrote of the organ's varied sounds. A physician had to learn by listening directly to a patient's chest.

The kissing bug disease tampers with this music, and doctors cannot explain why most people live with the parasite without any symptoms, while 20 to 30 percent of those infected suffer cardiac problems. To date, doctors cannot predict whose heart will be spared. Unless the infection is caught early, there is no cure. In a few infected people, like my auntie, the parasite strikes not the heart but the esophagus and the colon.

The Centers for Disease Control and Prevention (CDC) estimates that about three hundred thousand people with the kissing bug disease live in the United States. They are, like Tía Dora, immigrants. Close to six million people are currently infected, mostly in South America, Central America, and Mexico, and every year, more than ten thousand people die from the disease.

Tía Dora did not know these harrowing figures or that the parasite can be transmitted from a woman to her baby during pregnancy. In the United States, women are not routinely screened during pregnancy for the kissing bug disease, though each year more than three hundred babies may be born infected. My auntie also did not know that blood banks in the United States now screen people for the parasite the first time they donate. Fortunately, the disease does not spread like the common cold or Covid-19. Most people are infected from direct contact with a parasite-carrying kissing bug.

Formally called American trypanosomiasis, the disease is also known as Chagas after Carlos Chagas, the Brazilian doctor who discovered it in 1909 and was twice nominated for a Nobel Prize. The World Health Organization classifies Chagas as a neglected tropical disease. Others in that category include leprosy, sleeping sickness, and river blindness—afflictions the world has largely forgotten as they affect mainly poor people in countries beyond the borders of the United States and Western Europe.

The *New Yorker* has called the kissing bug disease the "red-headed stepchild" of vector-borne diseases—those caused when insects transmit pathogens—because even among the neglected, it has long been ignored.

...

I did not know any of this as a child. I only knew the hospital room that summer and Tía Dora with her pointy chin and the Spanish consonants in her mouth and how often the word Chagas made my mother sigh. I also knew that I wanted my auntie's love and suspected even then the impossibility of that desire.

IN SEARCH OF MY
FAMILY'S STORY

PALABRAS

In the seventies, Colombia's civil war remained tucked away in the mountains. Airplanes flew from Bogotá without exploding in the sky, and no one worried about being kidnapped for hefty ransoms. At the Palace of Justice, the Supreme Court judges, staffers, and cafeteria workers did not think of dying at the hands of the military or the rebels. All that would come later.

Tía Dora grew up with her parents—my grandparents—in Quiroga, a neighborhood on the south end of Bogotá. The houses looked like multicolored boxes stacked in the corner of a room, and the sidewalks curved toward stores that sold arepas, buñuelos, and glass bottles of Coca-Cola. The hills rose beyond the roofs, high and sepia-tinged, sprouting one-room homes constructed of wood and tar paper creating, at times, the impression that poor families were building in the direction of heaven. My abuelos, from the town of Ramiriquí, a few hours outside the capital, would probably have lived in the hills if it had not been for a government program that granted them a house in the city.

The family house had a front yard with two banana trees. A window in the living room looked out onto South Thirty-Third Street, and Tía Dora and my mother and their brothers and sisters—they were a family of eleven children—filled that living room over the years with gossip and a radio that played vallenato songs. The house had three bedrooms and accommodated itself to the size of the family. Beds were shared, pillows christened communal. Occasionally, another family rented a room so my grandparents, once farmers and now city folks without jobs, could earn extra cash. Behind the main house, rooms were built for two of my uncles and their wives and young children. The hens had their coop in the backyard, where they huddled in the cold and laid their generous eggs and, at night, surely dreamt of the campo.

The youngest of the girls, Tía Dora grew up on a merry-go-round of women's hands—of sisters, cousins, comadres, and cuñadas—and maybe, for that reason, she spent years referring to one of her oldest sisters as Mamá. Or perhaps Tía Dora knew the truth, knew exactly who her mother was, but loved her doting sister so much that she could think of no higher compliment than Mamá. As a child, she watched her older sisters make melcocha, a kind of molasses taffy. They heated the molasses, then waited for it to cool enough so they could pick it up and twist the melcocha into figure eights on the table, cut it into pieces, and hand it out to friends, primos, neighbors, whoever happened to walk by the front door.

Tía Dora had a predisposition toward joy. Her father's drinking did not bother her. She poured the cheap liquor down the drain and never blamed him. The sound of a brother coming home drunk at night and yelling at his wife pinched her ears. But men were men. They swung at each other and drank too much and still there they were.

Or maybe my auntie could afford to be generous since she planned to have a different future. By her late twenties, she was teaching elementary school children in the mornings, and in the evenings, working towards her bachelor's degree. She paid for the classes from her earnings, and she planned to be the primera: the first girl in the family to graduate from college. She carried herself as if she were made from copper, as if she was important, necessary even. One year, she saved her money to buy knee-high boots and Jackie O–style sunglasses. She gossiped with her cuñadas and nieces about men's faces. "Me encantan los hombres con bigotes," she'd say because she thought facial hair on a man delightful, though by all accounts she had no boyfriend.

...

The first time I met Tía Dora I was eight months old. My mother had been living in New Jersey six years by then, having left Colombia for work in the textile factories that dotted the towns along the Hudson River. She had been in the States long enough to marry a skinny Cuban exile, procure a green card, and give birth to me. She bundled me in a pink winter onesie, and we flew together from New York City to Bogotá, where Tía and the other aunties cradled me and changed my diaper and fed me formula. They had a crib ready for me, and over it they hung an enormous handmade doll with an obedient face and long braids the color of canela.

The second time we visited Colombia, I had acquired language. I was three. It was the summer of 1978, and Mami and I arrived in Bogotá to find Tía Dora embracing the fashion of the women's movement. She had cut her long wavy hair into a bob and wore blazers, a scarf around her neck. She looked like a woman who expected to work on Wall Street. Her handbag, thin and boxy, suggested a briefcase.

If the family stories are true, Tía Dora sat with me and the aunties one day, all of them chattering and laughing, and she decided to humor the other women, her older sisters and the cuñadas.

In Spanish, she whispered to me, "Say: puta."

I must have given her a dubious look. The word felt new to my ears, but she insisted. "Puta!" I cried to my mother and the aunties and the aunties married to my uncles.

My mouth latched on to the word. Puta, puta, puta. The word felt good and hard like carrying a knife between my teeth.

The women screamed in mock horror, then howled with laughter. I had called everyone in the room a whore.

...

If Tía were alive to read this, she would insist she never taught me vulgarities. "No fue así," she'd chide. "Fue una broma. You're making it sound so serious. It was funny."

But I was three and already negotiating with my auntie's ideas about language and transgression.

...

Tía Dora's sickness began with a swelling.

Around 1979, her belly inflated under the blouses she wore to teach at the local elementary school. She thought she was bloated.

She drank her mother's herbal teas. Nada. The discomfort persisted for a day, then another. Her belly stretched. In the shower, she would have looked down and seen it: her growing abdomen. Her brothers teased. They knew women who got knocked up. "Tell us! Who's the father?"

Tía Dora scowled, then laughed. She was not pregnant. She had barely kissed a man. She waved her brothers away. After another day or so, she ran a fever. The ice cubes melted on her forehead and the towels grew moist, soaking the heat from her body.

At the hospital in Bogotá, La Clínica Fray Bartolomé de las Casas, the nurse handed Tía Dora a baby-blue nightgown with a pattern of stars. A pain must have torn through her body. Tía turned to her sister and begged, "Pray the rosary for me."

The nurses looked at my auntie's belly. It was not the first time they had seen a woman pregnant and young, unmarried and terrified. They told Tía's sister that it was most likely an embarazo ectópico, the baby growing in her fallopian tubes.

In the hospital room, Tía Dora lay in bed, and her sister paid thirty pesos to have a rollaway bed brought in so she could stay the night. They recited the rosary together: Bendito es el fruto de tu vientre. Blessed is the fruit of your womb. Then, Tía Dora felt a chill. "Tengo frío," she said to her sister. "Give me my coat." She pointed at an empty chair. Her sister prayed harder. It was one thing to have a fever and another to lose your mind.

Gloved hands wheeled Tía Dora into an operating room. She might have kept her eyes open and watched the light above the nurse's face, the honey-tinted halo. She would have heard the instruments tinkling on the tray, the unwanted music of paper rustling, latex gloves snapping into place, the hum of orders being issued. She could not have heard the blade, its silver face pressing into her belly.

After the exploratory surgery, the doctors told her sister, "Tiene los intestinos de diez personas." My auntie's large intestine had dilated, widened, begun to go loose inside her body. She had enough of a large intestine for ten people. The doctors offered a colostomy bag. It would get her through her last year of college, and when she graduated, a colostomy bag hung from the side of her belly. The doctors believed she might live a year, maybe two. No one suspected a parasite.

. . .

The women in my family decided to save Tía Dora. That is not how they told the story later. They credited the men: one particular doctor and also the husband of another auntie who knew of a clinic in Manhattan for poor people. But it is clear that my mother and my aunties made a decision: Tía Dora would not die. They shipped colostomy bags to Colombia. They paid for her flight to the United States in the winter of 1980. They asked my father if he would be so kind as to pick up Tía Dora at JFK.

In the car that night on the way to the airport, my father's skinny fingers gripped the steering wheel. A Cuban, he had curly hair and bushy eyebrows, and he wore a flannel button-down shirt under a thin jacket. He was a man who refused winter. Now, he was also irritated, tense, and short-tempered probably because he felt nervous, afraid even. Driving made him uncomfortable. The responsibility of it frustrated him.

My mother sat next to him, a rag doll of a woman, and like a muñeca, she was consistent and quiet. Papi, a jack-in-the-box, grumbled about the traffic and why we had not left earlier and did Mami have money for the tolls, but like a doll, my mother was steady in her moods—her half smile, her nonjudgment. She answered his questions and looked out the window at the black road ahead of her.

I was five years old, and my mother had stuffed me into a coat so heavy and snowball-resistant that my arms could move only up and down. The mittens on my hands were as puffy as pillows. But I was enjoying having the back seat to myself. My sister, Liliana, had stayed home with someone. She was still new, only four months old, and I did not quite understand that she was a permanent addition to our family. The world had always been as it was at that moment in the car: the rag doll and the jack-in-the-box and me.

I was the only one thrilled about the drive. I loved airports. I loved the balloons people brought for those who arrived and the flowers too. I loved running around the grown-ups, squeezing between their bodies. I loved how people hollered the names of sisters and cousins, and how they cried and hugged. Every arrival was a premio, a prize someone deserved.

My mother hated the airport.

Two years earlier, on our way back from Colombia, agents at JFK had opened our bags. The men picked through my mother's panties and socks. They tasted the arequipe and the hard candies too. Later, she complained to her sister: "¡Hasta los pañales!" Even the diapers were suspect.

At the airport that night, my mother worried that the immigration men would not let Tía Dora through, and so while I ran around the waiting area, Mami stood with my father and all the women and men, everyone in winter coats and heavy scarves, and monitored the doors and tried not to think of the worst. She watched sisters and abuelas and couples arrive, but no Tía Dora. Maybe they had detained her. Maybe she'd gotten sick during the flight. Maybe they had simply refused her entry.

The crowd thinned. My father grew irritable. Where was she? He still had to drive us all back home, and it was the middle of December and the roads just awful.

The doors opened again. Tía Dora took a tentative step out, and the corners of my mother's lips collapsed. Her sister's face had thinned. How much weight had she lost? Already, she looked like a young woman about to die.

...

In the back seat of the car, Tía and I studied each other. I did not have my mother's worry. I did not know that grown women could become sick and die. If anyone had asked, I would have said my auntie looked like all the grown women I knew except she was flaca. Also, someone in Colombia had stuffed her into a ruana and coat. I sensed a kindred spirit. An auntie who did not get to dress herself. An auntie who was coming to live in our apartment in Union City, New Jersey.

...

In Colombia, Tía Dora had her mother, three sisters, and several cuñadas. In Jersey, she had my mother and Tía Rosa who

14

my father eventually nicknamed Radio Auntie since this auntie talked all the time. Radio Auntie had a bundle of hair that looked like black cotton on top of her head. She was the oldest auntie in Jersey, the one who had no children of her own but whom Tía Dora had once called Mamá.

Over the next six months, Radio Auntie ushered Tía Dora onto buses and subways. She and my mother fed her papas rellenas. They learned that Columbia-Presbyterian Medical Center in Manhattan had specific days and times when any patient would be seen, regardless of whether the person could pay. They shuttled Tía Dora across the Hudson River to the hospital. They helped her get in and out of the hospital gown and met with Dr. Alfred M. Markowitz. The surgeon had strong eyebrows and thinning silver hair carefully groomed away from his face. He looked crisp and alert in his suit underneath his white coat, the kind of man that made you think of a clean piece of paper.

The doctors in Colombia had not suspected the kissing bug disease but Dr. Markowitz did. In an article in the *New York Times*, years after his death, he was celebrated as an old-school physician-teacher who quizzed his residents, on the spot, about obscure medical conditions. This may explain how Dr. Markowitz diagnosed Tía Dora with the disease, because only in a few number of cases does the parasite attack the gastrointestinal system, making it so that the large intestine begins to lose its shape. Food starts to collect in the colon. The person's belly begins to swell. A man can, as Tía Dora did, appear pregnant. Without intervention, toxins can seep from the intestines and kill the person.

Dr. Markowitz explained that Tía Dora would need several abdominal surgeries. My mother, anxious and worried, asked how much it would cost. In Colombia, if you didn't have health insurance, you had to save your earnings before a doctor would perform a procedure. "We'll have to raise the money," Mami said quickly, imagining the expense, and she thought about asking a local Spanish radio station to make the announcement that our family needed many thousands of dollars to save my auntie's life.

"Don't worry about the cost," the doctor said.

The women in my family did not know how hospitals took care of patients who did not have insurance. They did not know about Medicaid. They did not know the phrase *indigent patients*. They believed the doctor himself would pay for the surgeries. They insisted our family had been blessed.

...

In New Jersey, my mother and Radio Auntie and Tía Dora made audio recordings for my grandmother in Colombia. Tía told her mother about the doctor and the nurses and the hospital but didn't mention an interpreter. She had studied English and apparently understood more than she could speak. Or maybe no one needs an interpreter when a priest comes to offer last rites.

"I got scared," she whispered into the cassette recording, describing the day of her first surgery, but she did not lose faith, she assured her mother. Then, Dr. Markowitz came to her room. "He spoke to me in such a sensitive way. All in English."

He wanted to be clear with her. "I am asking for luck for you and for me," he said. "If I make a mistake in any way, I ask for forgiveness."

She assured him that he possessed all her forgiveness, all her gratitude.

So many doctors filled the operating room that Tía Dora lost count of them. Some were residents. One a cardiologist. Another an anesthesiologist. And then she was asleep and the men busy slicing open her belly.

When she woke from the first surgery, Tía spoke in English. She meant to say that she wanted to see Dr. Markowitz, but "Por favor, quiero ver el Dr. Markowitz!" collapsed in the translation, and she cried, "Please I like Dr. Markowitz!" She cried it repeatedly until he appeared and clasped her hands.

THE APPLE

Tía Dora spent a month hospitalized at Columbia-Presbyterian Medical Center. Her birthday that July fell on a Sunday. "I told them I wanted to go to church." Her cardiologist had to sign off on the venture, though she was traveling no farther than the hospital chapel by way of a wheelchair.

The doctors monitored her closely. When her fever spiked, Tía explained that ice would bring it down quickly. "We have to find the cause," one of the doctors said. If they discovered it, however, Tía did not record it for her mother. Neither did she mention a parasite or a kissing bug. Instead, she narrated her body, how after the first surgery she looked down and saw the horrifying scar across her lower abdomen. "I almost fainted." She turned to Dr. Markowitz, who was probably very proud of the precision of his surgical work, and said, "Please, doctor. It's ugly. It's terrible."

The surgeon smiled kindly and promised that he would make it better with the next surgery.

One day, still in the hospital, Tía Dora began to cry and could not stop. A nurse rang Dr. Markowitz. Tía Dora told him, "I want to see . . ." and she had a long list of women, all of whom were in

Colombia. Her mother, her aunties, her sisters. Yes, Radio Auntie came to visit her, but she worked for long stretches of hours as a home health aide, and my mother lived all the way over in Jersey with two young girls.

The son of Jewish immigrants, Dr. Markowitz apparently knew as much about the need for the mother tongue as he did about neglected diseases and the gastrointestinal system. "It's normal," Dr. Markowitz told Tía about her longing for home. But she could not leave, not yet. He penned a note to the Colombian embassy in New York City, explaining that she needed to stay in the United States for further medical care, including one or two more surgeries.

He made no mention of Tía Dora's immigration status. Perhaps he didn't ask. Perhaps he didn't care. Perhaps he didn't want to know that Tía Dora had overstayed her tourist visa, that she was, as we say in Spanish, sin papeles, undocumented.

...

When Tía Dora returned home to us between surgeries, I belted out the nursery rhymes I was learning at Holy Family Roman Catholic School. I sang to her about farmers taking wives and a rat taking the cheese. Everyone in the nursery rhyme was grabbing what did not belong to them, even the nurse, and then one afternoon the hospital arranged for a nurse to visit Tía in our living room.

Our home was a first-floor apartment in Union City. The neighborhood reminded Tía of Quiroga, her neighborhood in Bogotá. "At times I forget that I'm sick," she told her mother in a recording. The women in our building spoke Spanish and dropped by with rice dishes and wanted to know how Tía Dora felt and told her she looked good. Everyone agreed on this: she looked good. She looked better than when she had arrived from Colombia.

Maybe the nurse took a bus to reach our apartment and marched through the streets with her medical bag swinging against her hip. She would have passed the shop where the Cuban women rolled tobacco, the bakeries that sold señoritas—with their perfect layers of vanilla custard—and the discount store where women's panties filled the wooden bins. Maybe those stores came later. It was 1981. In a few years Union City would have its first Cuban mayor, Robert Menendez, and the newspapers would report what Tía Dora and I could already see: outside of Miami, our town had the most Cubans in the United States.

Settling into the sofa, Tía Dora and the nurse nodded at each other. My mother sensed that the nurse had questions. Of course she had questions. My mother called for me to stop singing about farmers and to help translate for my auntie.

"Let's check your blood pressure," the nurse said to Tía.

My auntie rolled up her sleeves. She still wore the escapulario, the Catholic necklace with its two square pieces of cloth that mimick a monk's garments and are supposed to bring good luck. A hospital nurse had given it to her.

The nurse unhooked a stethoscope from her bag and asked, "How are you feeling today?"

"Good," Tía Dora whispered.

My auntie looked at me. The nurse followed her eyes.

I was six and still had short ponytails. No one said, "Your auntie has a disease that could kill her." No one said, "Your auntie needs you." They didn't have to. It was obvious from the way the nurse said, "Tell your aunt . . ." and the way Tía Dora told me, "Dile a la enfermera . . ."

The nurse inspected the skin where the colostomy bag was attached to Tía's body and looked for signs of infection. She had questions for me and directions too. No one cared that I was only about to start first grade. I knew both languages or enough. I was my auntie's ears and her tongue, and when I did not know a word, I stitched the English noun to Spanish verbs, and Tía Dora beamed at me as if I were the smartest girl alive.

...

For years after the surgeries, I did not think of Tía Dora as a woman with a serious illness. She was my skinny tía, the tía with scars on her belly, the tía who had several surgeries over the course of a year and then continued to live with my parents, sister, and me. I thought of her as the auntie whose belly hurt her some days, who couldn't always eat when she wanted, who was, as Mami said, delicada.

The illness then was a part of Tía like her brown eyelashes. At least that is what I believed. When I turned thirteen, however, one of the older tías, Auntie Biblia, came to live with us and told me the truth.

...

It was 1988, and my parents had moved us to our own house a few miles north of Union City. The kitchen looked like a garden.

The wallpaper boasted rows of green apples and pears with leafy stems. The refrigerator was a giant potato stuffed into a rincón under the staircase, and the pressure cooker whistled every Saturday before noon: a fat bird sitting high in the trees. One window faced the long driveway in front and the other a quiet alley behind the house. Our house, with its kitchen-garden, was probably the oldest one on our block, but it was ours.

One Saturday afternoon, the kitchen-garden held nine of us: my parents, three aunties, two auntie husbands, my baby sister, and me. Tía Dora sat at the table. My mother fried patacones. Another auntie poured soda, and one of the auntie husbands stood at the threshold to the kitchen, holding the doorframe, as if he had installed it. The table did not have enough chairs for everyone to sit and eat at the same time so we took turns at the table, and the grown ups complained in Spanish about the wars in Central America and the price of meat in Union City.

My mother, her short hair dyed a shade of auburn, leaned against the stove. "What they're charging for a pound of chuletas is . . ." Her voice trailed. The oil sizzled in the pan. She searched for the right word and found it: "It's barbaric."

Her older sister, María de Jesus, whom a cousin later called La Biblia, the Bible, on account of her long memory, refused to be outdone. "It's worse at the supermarket on Palisade," she retorted.

Radio Auntie added that the price of eggs was worse still. Maybe she eyed her husband. The man could eat a dozen eggs by himself in one sitting.

The television in the next room blared with news of the dead in El Salvador. My father, who had fought against Fidel Castro's army in Cuba, sat in the kitchen by the window, listening. He was turning fifty that year but still looked like the lanky soldier I saw once in a photograph from when he was nineteen. He heard about the dead in El Salvador and turned to the auntie husbands and said, "Qué mierda." The men agreed. Wars were shit.

Tía Dora wore a knee-length billowy skirt and a blouse a tad wider than her thin shoulders. Her three sisters complained that she was nothing but huesos. They were round women themselves: moons, globes, oval dresser mirrors. Tía Dora was a candlestick. She had thin fingers, a long nose, brazos delgados. She dyed her hair a light brown and once a shade of blonde that had looked like a yellow flame on her head. She floated through the kitchen-garden, her hair shaped into the voluminous curls popular that season.

My mother tried to get Tía Dora to eat. Here's a bowl of soup. A plate of pescado. A baked potato with nothing on it.

"No, mi vida," Tía Dora said. "No puedo."

"It's only a little," my mother insisted.

Tía shook her head and pressed her palm to her belly. "I can't," she murmured and sighed at the baked fish as if it were a man she could never love.

Later that evening, the house emptied of aunties and auntie husbands. The sun turned into a brassy light at the bedroom window on the second floor. Auntie Biblia perched next to me on the twin bed, the mattress sagging under our weight.

She looked at me as if I were a book she had already read. In Colombia, Auntie Biblia had taught elementary school children in villages how to read and sweep the dirt floors of their one-room homes. In Jersey, she told me stories about communist rebels who longed to become literate and girls who could never escape the violence of their fathers' hands.

In a hushed tone, Auntie Biblia said, "Dora está enferma, pero muy enferma."

I leaned in. The way she talked about Tía's illness sounded strange to me, as if there had been another option. But Tía Dora had always had nurses and doctors, always needed naps and special attention. It was normal.

"Dora almost died in Colombia—that's how sick she was," Auntie Biblia said.

"What happened to her?"

"She ate an apple."

I didn't argue. I was thirteen. Like everyone else, I had read the Bible. I knew what happened to women who tasted fruit they were forbidden to touch.

...

I pinned Auntie Biblia's story to the one I knew best—the story of Eve's transgression in the Garden of Eden, her subsequent exile and punishment. Or maybe it had nothing to do with that most famous of stories. I had gotten my first period and I was beginning to understand that every woman is two women, herself and her body. Or maybe, as the child of immigrant women—the daughter, the niece, la sobrina—I was required to have a relationship with fiction. *She ate an apple and almost died.* Migration and poverty swallowed parts of the story, made it so the stories were half-told, almost perdidos. Once upon a time, Tía Dora ate an apple in Colombia, and that was why she was sick in New Jersey.

BICHOS

Auntie Biblia's stories, akin to praying the rosary, repeated. She moved about our kitchen table with her pomegranate lipstick and her tall tales about Colombia's beauty pageants and priests who wanted more than limosna, her story about how Tía Dora had almost died, that's how sick she was.

I might have been almost fifteen when the kitchen-garden started to feel crowded for my arms and legs, my new height, which at five feet two inches felt quite tall. I could see stains on the wallpaper.

Thinking about Tía Dora, I asked, "How could eating a fruit almost kill her?"

"It was contaminated," Auntie Biblia answered, matter-of-fact.

"How?"

"A bicho. The fruit was contaminated by a bicho."

...

Bicho is a Spanish word for insect. It can also mean a man's penis, and in some parts of Latin America, a little devil.

It did not surprise me that a bicho tried to kill Tía Dora because my mother waged a furious war in our kitchen-garden against roaches. One time, Mami opened a cupboard, spotted a cockroach, took off her house slipper, and flicked the roach from the cupboard to the kitchen floor, where she smashed it repeatedly with her slippered foot, then scooped it up into a dustpan and hauled it to the trash bin.

The killing tired my mother. Sweat gathered on her forehead, and her body looked heavier, sadder. Still, she battled.

By the time I heard about Tía Dora and the bicho, I already knew I was no match for anything that creeped and crawled, whether it was an insect out in the wild or a pest in the kitchen. When I opened the utensil drawer to find a cockroach, its splayed antennae poking out from under a stack of forks as if it were ready to fight me, I slammed the drawer shut and almost threw up.

Tía Dora hated bichos, too. Watching my mother squish a roach on the stovetop with a paper towel, Tía grimaced, then closed her eyes, as if the mere sight of the cucaracha offended her sensibilities. When she peeked in my mother's direction, she said, "Ay, mi vida," as if it pained her that my sweet mother had to do such work. I had already fled to the other side of the room and did not move again until the cockroach was officially dead, its six legs cracked.

It was not that Tía and I were special. Some women could kill a cockroach, and some, like Tía and me, could not. Auntie Biblia shook her head sadly at the two of us. She smashed cockroaches without comment. She had seen worse. When Tía Dora was not around to hear, she told me a bicho had come after another auntie in Colombia. "Her name was Margarita," Auntie Biblia said.

"Who was she?"

"Tío Guillermo's wife. She had Chagas too."

My auntie didn't talk about a parasite, only a bicho, and how after Tía Margarita was infected, her heart turned into a rock inside her chest. "She had to sleep sitting up." Otherwise her heart, so heavy, so much a piedra, suffocated her. She had five grown children, and her last one, a boy, was only a baby when the doctors realized the bicho had gotten her.

No one knew why the doctors in Colombia diagnosed Tía Margarita with the kissing bug disease but not Tía Dora. Maybe doctors were like bichos: a matter of chance.

One day, the stories about Tía Margarita stopped.

"What happened to her?" I asked Auntie Biblia.

"She died."

...

The aunties and my mother did not speak to me about public health policies and the mechanics of capitalism. They did not explain that the roaches in our kitchen had to do with the working-class town where we lived and with not wanting to pay for a monthly fumigator. They did not know that kissing bugs are usually found in warm, rural areas in South America, Central America, and Mexico, in houses made from branches and mud and the fronds of palm trees. That only certain species of kissing bugs carry the parasite that causes the disease.

Instead the women in my family constructed a private mythology. While other girls my age were taught to fear rabid dogs and horrible men, I learned to be terrified of an insect the size of my fingernail, an insect that could kill a woman's heart. And as with all private mythologies, this one began before my mother was born.

...

Peeling an orange one day in the kitchen, when it was only the two of us, Auntie Biblia said, "Pobrecita la Linda. My mother suffered so much."

"Who's Linda?" I asked.

"The girl who died."

"What girl?"

"Your grandmother's daughter. She died when she was only two. Worms got her. One day, the worms just started coming out of her nose, and she died. Poor girl."

Auntie Biblia said the gusanos dropped from Linda's nose, spilling onto the ground, coiling and wriggling. My grandmother wailed. Neighbor women hoisted the toddler away from the pile of worms, but it was no use. She died. Auntie Biblia never used the word "disease," and I never learned what worms Linda had.

This happened when my family still lived hours from Bogotá, in Ramiriquí, a town that looks today as the Spaniards constructed it in the 1500s: a square ringed by a stone church and local government offices and houses with second-story balconies. The year Linda died, the women in Ramiriquí still monitored each other's movements, their marriages and children. When my grandmother gave birth to my mother a year or so after Linda's death, the women in the town told her, "Dios te la mandó." God sent her to you.

Linda was the tía I did not get to have. The tía who died before she could become a tía. Because she died, my oldest tías took precautions with my mother. They chased my mother around the house and out of the house and forced the purgante down her throat, determined to prevent the worms from getting her. The medication worked. Mami survived the worms.

...

These stories pinched my heart every time I heard them. Worms could fall from a child's nose. A woman's own heart could kill her, and no doctor could stop it. Still, without realizing it, I was writing a myth too, an American one. If anyone had suggested that Tía Dora might die one day from the kissing bug disease, I would have said, "Don't be ridiculous. We have the best doctors and hospitals and medicine." As long as my auntie stayed here with us, she would never die.

...

Years later, when I started reading about kissing bugs, I did not know what I would find, but I absolutely did not expect to come across Charles Darwin.

In 1835, Darwin was twenty-six and four years into his trip through South America—the one that gave him the basis for his book *On the Origin of Species*. In March 1835, he and his guide rode mules through the plains of Argentina. The land was flat and the air hot, and for a full day, Darwin found no water and only a few houses. When they neared the village of Luján de Cuyo, he noticed a field the color of blood. A locust invasion. People raced from their cottages and set branches on fire and waved the torched bark at the locusts. They shouted, hoping the noise and smoke would turn away the tiny beasts, but nothing worked. Darwin rode on.

The men had ten mules with them, and when they all finally escaped the locusts and reached Luján de Cuyo, Darwin expected to sleep well. The village was nestled among gardens. It boasted a river and rows of poplars and willows. Who doesn't sleep like a king under a willow tree?

But when Darwin closed his eyes that night in Argentina, the kissing bugs crept out from their hiding places, and the insects did not care if it was Charles Darwin or not. The sun had vanished. Ravenous, they set off for the evening, creeping onto his body. They expected him to be asleep. They expected to feed on him. But Darwin was awake and horrified, and later, despite being a man of science, he wrote how "disgusting" it was to feel all these bichos "nearly an inch long & black & soft crawling in all parts of your person—gorged with your blood."

...

In 1959, nearly eight decades after his death, doctors began debating whether Darwin had suffered the kissing bug disease. He was certainly sick for most of his life, after his epic trip to South America, and in the quest for a diagnosis, doctors and others have speculated that he could have had any one of more than forty conditions including malaria, arsenic poison, Crohn's disease, psychosomatic illnesses, lactose intolerance, and the kissing bug disease. The only fact we know for sure from Darwin's notebooks is that he met face to face with kissing bugs in

Argentina and Chile. Today, the insects would be classified as *Triatoma infestans.*

In Chile, the kissing bug was "flat as a wafer," Darwin wrote. It was starving. An officer offered to let the insect bite him. Darwin watched as the kissing bug charged, plunging a needle from its mouth, a proboscis, into the man's finger, stabbing his flesh. Permitted to feast, the insect did so for ten minutes, growing to five, maybe six times its own size. It turned as fat as a grape.

Darwin stored the insect along with his other specimens. Eighteen days later, it wanted to feed again. Darwin refused it, and he and his servant, Syms Covington, kept meticulous notes. How long could a kissing bug live from a single feeding of a man's finger? Four and half months. "A most bold and fearless insect," Darwin finally observed in his notebook.

In the 1500s, three hundred years before Darwin traveled through South America, the Spanish soldier Gerónimo de Bibar also noticed the kissing bugs in Chile. He wrote that they have a fondness for warm temperatures and "sting very badly."

...

In 1855, twenty years after Charles Darwin encountered the kissing bugs in South America, the entomologist John Lawrence LeConte traveled across the United States documenting some five thousand species of beetles and found a species of the kissing bug in Georgia. He named it *Conorhinus sanguisuga* and kept detailed notes about the insect (it had hairy legs). "It is remarkable," LeConte wrote, ". . . for sucking the blood of mammals, particularly of children." Once bitten, the children developed welts on their skin that sometimes persisted for a year.

Kissing bugs came to be called triatomine insects and classified in the family of assassin bugs, or Reduviidae, for their vampire-like tendencies. All over the Americas, though, people adopted other names. In Texas and the Southwest, people have called the kissing bug a bloodsucker, and in Argentina and Bolivia, people say it's a vinchuca, a word that probably comes from Quechua, a language millions of people speak today in South America and that dates back to the Inca Empire. Vinchuca means "bug that lets itself fall" and is probably a reference to how kissing bugs slip out from the crevices in the walls of mud houses, falling toward the bodies of their sleeping victims.

In Central America and Mexico, people say the kissing bug is a chinche, a name also used for bedbugs. Years after I had grown up and left home, a man from Mexico tried to explain it to me this way: there are little chinches and big chinches. The kissing bug, he told me, is a big chinche.

...

I did not grow up hearing any nicknames for triatomine insects. We didn't even use the word pito, which is what Colombians call the kissing bug. In our family, the only word we had for the kissing bug was the same one we used for every other nasty insect: bicho.

And we certainly did not know that at the end of the nineteenth century, the kissing bug was almost named for a Black man in Washington, DC.

...

It began when an elderly man woke up in DC one hot June morning in 1899 and found his nose and his cheeks swollen to such grotesque proportions that he couldn't open his eyes properly. In the emergency room, doctors figured a bug must have bitten him during the night. Had the man seen an insect? No. Another man dashed to the same hospital with his upper lip puffed up like a baseball painted the color of rubies. No, he had not seen a bug or felt a bite. Other patients arrived in the same condition—their upper lips inflated into startling red balloons.

A *Washington Post* reporter began following the mystery bug bites. "In the absence of a scientific name for the creature," he wrote, "it has been suggested to name it Dorseyfoultz, on account of the skill and persistence with which it evades observation and defies capture." That summer, Dorsey Foultz, a Black man, had eluded local police who wanted him on murder charges. The reporter apparently did not find it problematic to name a potentially dangerous insect after a Black man. Despite the article in the *Washington Post*, the name did not stick, probably because news of the bug bites was spreading beyond DC and no one outside of the district had heard of the suspect.

People began arriving that summer at emergency rooms in other cities with terrible bug bites. In New York City, Bellevue Hospital admitted six people and Boston alone had a dozen cases. One Delaware newspaper reported that kissing bugs were attacking policemen on duty. In Washington, DC, men with bandaged faces begged for scraps and coins, claiming that the bug had attacked them and they could no longer work.

The patient narratives repeated: an insect appeared, usually near dusk, sometimes later in the night. The victim didn't see it, only felt the bite to the mouth, and then the insect fled. By morning the person's lip had swollen.

Newspapers named the mysterious insect the kissing bug. What else to call a little devil that only wanted to suck on a person's mouth?

Then the reports of deaths began to appear. In Philadelphia, a six-year-old boy woke on a Tuesday morning with his face swollen and a "purple spot" over his lip. Two days later he was dead, and the kissing bug blamed. A two-year-old girl died in Trenton days after her mother noticed bug bites on her legs. In Chicago, a doctor wrote "kissing bug" as the cause of one woman's death. The doctor had not seen the bicho, but his patient, Mary Steger, had died at the age of thirty-three with an injured lip. Chicago's health officials, however, handed the death certificate back to the doctor. Take it to the coroner, they told him. He did. The city coroner examined Steger's body. Her face was badly swollen, and the bruise still appeared on the woman's lip. The coroner concluded that she had blood poisoning, but he could not say for sure what had killed her. Maybe it was a kissing bug.

Warnings about kissing bugs appeared in newspapers as far away as El Paso and Las Vegas. Newspapers did not include drawings of the swollen faces. The terror pivoted towards the possibility of the lips deformed, the human face unmade. One entomologist insisted that the insect bit people on the mouth because it found the movement of human lips "irritating." A doctor proposed that it was probably a "nervous disorder" which had nothing to do with insects, and in Washington, DC, a man penned a letter to a local paper, arguing that the kissing bugs were innocent. The giant, swollen lips, he wrote, were due to "the excessive eating of strawberries."

Not all reactions were serious. Shopkeepers sold kissing bug jewelry. Poets wrote lyrical odes to the insect. The *Chicago Daily Tribune* ran a story on how to craft a mock kissing bug from wire and paper for the purpose of eliciting "feminine shrieks."

Leland Ossian Howard, the head of entomology at the US Department of Agriculture, finally addressed the issue in a paper published in *Popular Science Monthly*, explaining that the bites could be from six different insects. The one best known to entomologists, he observed, was the "ferocious" insect called the "blood-sucking cone-nose," usually found in the southern and western states. It bit people everywhere: on the arms and legs and feet. It was the insect LeConte had identified a few decades before. But Howard argued that the bites during the summer of 1899 were a matter of mass hysteria inflated by the media. He did not explain why some people had died after the bug bites.

The summer ended. The stories vanished. Then, more than a decade later, in the early twentieth century, news arrived from Brazil. The "blood-sucking cone-nose" insects there had been found to carry a parasite that could kill the human heart. Newspapermen evidently didn't remember the name bloodsuckers or even "cone-nose." They turned to their archives, it seems, found the stories from 1899, and christened the insect the "kissing bug."

DR. CHAGAS

By the time I turned sixteen, Tía Dora had started watching wrestling matches on television. She sank into the sofa one day, her thin body under a ruana, and cheered for what looked to me like a long line of bulky men in Speedos and capes. "Qué cuerpo que tiene el hombre," she said almost breathless. What a body the man has.

She looked at me with an expectant face until I finally said, "They're big guys."

Satisfied, she turned back to watch Hulk Hogan waving at the crowds. I picked at my fingernail and said, "All they do is hurt each other."

"No, they know what they're doing," she said with confidence and without taking her eyes off the television, where Hulk Hogan's giant mustache almost filled the screen.

I thought about language and how even these white men did not choose their words but had, if the news accounts were true, been given scripts. Their words had been orchestrated and also their pain and their bodies, and so they flew across the stage, bruising each other to the cheers of the audience at Madison Square Garden and my Colombian auntie in Jersey. At the end of the show, the men left the stage, their bodies intact. Only decades later would we read the reports of professional wrestlers with brain injuries. It was akin to the kissing bug disease. You did not see the body in ruins at first.

Tía Dora never called her illness the kissing bug disease. It was always Chagas and sometimes El Chagas. It occurred to me that the word might have its own story. Tía had several dictionaries. Maybe she knew. "Why is it called Chagas?" I asked her.

"It was the name of the man who discovered it."

The news stung. I had thought the name might be Latin in origin and refer to the body being ripped apart by a bicho or that it might be a kind of stage name, like Hulk Hogan, whose real first name was Terry. But Chagas was the name of an actual man, and when I learned this, the story of what had happened to Tía Dora grew legs. I imagined the man, this doctor, in South America. I decided that he was still alive. He was a man with black eyes, strolling the streets in Bogotá or maybe in Buenos Aires or Rio de Janeiro or Havana. Later, when I begin to read about the disease, I found that he had, in fact, been born in Brazil at a time when everything people knew about infectious diseases and bichos was changing.

...

At the end of the nineteenth century the superpowers cracked the world into pieces—the United States snatched Cuba, Puerto Rico, and the Philippines, and Britain and other European nations grabbed most of Africa. Building an empire meant encountering pathogens transmitted by insects and the diseases they caused: yellow fever, malaria, sleeping sickness. At times, the colonial powers used these illnesses as a reason for invasions like in 1898 when US politicians, newspapers, and the surgeon general argued that battling yellow fever required seizing control of Cuba. It was also during this time that the British started two schools, one in London and the other in Liverpool, devoted to a field they called "tropical medicine." Some doctors served the medical needs of white British families; others focused on the diseases of the empire, which these doctors associated with Black and Brown bodies.

Physicians thought that contaminated air called miasma made a person sick—-that malaria, cholera, and other diseases came about and were transmitted when rotting matter generated polluted air. By the 1890s, though, they had embraced germ theory. Louis Pasteur showed the world that living microorganisms existed and caused fermentation. Robert Koch demonstrated that bacteria leads to tuberculosis. And when Ronald Ross determined that the *Anopheles* mosquito carts around the parasite for malaria, insects in the colonies came under suspicion.

No one knew at the time that kissing bugs were guilty, that they carry in their guts the parasite *Trypanosoma cruzi*, that this parasite is found only in the Americas but has a cousin, so to speak, in West and Central Africa called *Trypanosoma brucei gambiense*. The *T. b. gambiense* parasite jumps from tsetse flies to humans, sneaking into a person's central nervous system and causing human African trypanosomiasis, or sleeping sickness, a disease that left untreated leads to paranoia, coma, and ultimately death. The disease killed more than a quarter of a million people in Uganda in five years at the start of the twentieth century, and because it threatened the supply of rubber and ivory from Africa to Europe, Belgium and Britain declared war on the parasite during those years. The London School of Tropical Medicine made sleeping sickness the focus of its research agenda. The Liverpool School of Tropical Medicine sent a team of scientists to the Congo and Uganda. By 1908, a Sleeping Sickness Bureau opened in London, and when international conferences convened to discuss the matter of this deadly parasite, all the imperial powers arrived: Belgium, France, Germany, and Italy.

It is strange to think of it this way, but Tía Dora was battling a parasite whose cousin tried to take down the European empires before the First World War.

...

By the start of the twentieth century, Brazil, like other countries at the time, was contending with a number of diseases in its port cities: malaria, yellow fever, the bubonic plague. It waged a public health campaign in Rio de Janeiro for several years, mostly vanquishing yellow fever and establishing a state-of the-art research lab known today as the Oswaldo Cruz Institute. In 1907, when the Central Railroad Company began installing tracks in the countryside, hours north of Rio, and workers contracted malaria, they reached out to the institute, which sent them Dr. Carlos Chagas. In his late twenties and only four years out of medical school, the young doctor had already gone after malaria in São Paulo and had succeeded in bringing it under control.

In pictures, Dr. Chagas is almost as skinny as Tía Dora. He has a nose so long it drags the rest of his face into a state of melancholy. Or it could be his eyebrows. They dip at the end, making his face look longer, más serio, than most. His mustache is perfectly groomed. He wears a shirt with a starched high collar tightly buttoned under his chin and a thin tie that makes him look more flaco, but also compact and efficient.

Leaving Rio de Janeiro in 1907, Dr. Chagas may have passed through the city's business district. Its streets had been paved and widened recently to resemble Paris. The new buildings gleamed in the sunlight: the National Library, the Monroe Palace, the Municipal Theater. The battle against yellow fever had served as the pretext for destroying the old homes and businesses on these streets and erecting the new Parisian-style buildings. Starting in 1902, health inspectors began barging into the homes of poor families in Rio, searching for possible breeding grounds for mosquitoes linked to yellow fever. When inspectors declared homes unsanitary, city officials slated the apartments for demolition and pushed out the families. But it did not happen without resistence. In 1903, one group of neighbors protested the displacement by throwing stones at health inspectors until the men left.

On the train that day, Dr. Chagas slept and maybe dreamt of small monkeys. The train pushed on for another two days, reaching a part of the country so rich in iron ore that it was called General Mines. He arrived in the town of Lassance, where the main street ran parallel to the train tracks. There was dust and heat and horses. The men had named one street after knives and another after gunshots. There was a brothel and bars for drinking, but also families who lived in homes with walls made of mud.

Dr. Chagas set up his office in a train car and began implementing anti-malaria measures. After the outbreak was under control, he spent another year traveling ahead of the railroad construction, looking for possible malaria hotspots. One day, an engineer pointed to an insect the workers called "the barber" for the way it sucked blood from them at night while they slept. In those days, barbers performed minor medical procedures including bloodletting. The barber insect was a kissing bug known today as *Panstronglyus megistus,* and when Dr. Chagas sliced it open and examined the insect's digestive tract under a microscope, he saw a parasite, a trypanosome, like the one that causes sleeping sickness in Africa. He shipped several kissing bugs to the lab in Rio, where his mentor had the insects feed on monkeys. The animals became infected with the parasite and later died. Dr. Chagas named the parasite *Trypanosoma cruzi* after his mentor, Oswaldo Cruz.

In the spring of 1909, Dr. Chagas took blood samples from people in Lassance: men, women, children. He found evidence of *T. cruzi,* but the people were healthy. In one house, where he had discovered an infected cat, however, he witnessed kissing bugs bite a two-year-old girl named Berenice. Two or three weeks later, when Dr. Chagas returned to the house, the girl was running a fever. Dr. Chagas began to examine her. The toddler's face was bloated, her skin waxy. He pressed his hands to her belly and rib cage. Her spleen and liver were swollen.

Berenice's mother must have held the feverish child so that Dr. Chagas could stick the syringe in her arm for a blood sample. The child would have cried and stared in horror at the man with the mustache.

Back in his boxcar, probably somewhat anxiously, Dr. Chagas placed a slide with Berenice's blood under the microscope and peered into the lens. He saw the culprit magnified: *T. cruzi.* The parasite that had killed small monkeys in the lab in Rio was here circulating in the body of this sick child. The parasite resembled the one that causes human African trypanosomiasis. He named the disease American trypanosomiasis.

It was a heady moment for Dr. Chagas and by extension for Brazil's medical and scientific community. All sorts of serious white men were hunting deadly microbes around the world, and here in Brazil, Dr. Chagas had found a parasite no one knew existed. But while he could link *T. cruzi* to fever in a toddler and the deaths of laboratory animals, he could not prove that the parasite led to severe illness.

. . .

The men who chased after the pathogens causing yellow fever, malaria, and sleeping sickness already knew what damage these diseases could inflict on the human body—the body on fire in the case of malaria, the mind taken hostage in the case of sleeping sickness. These germ hunters knew the illness and set out to find the complicit parasites, bacteria and viruses. Dr. Chagas had discovered the parasite and proven that in the lab it could kill marmosets and guinea pigs, but he was not sure, early on, about the parasite's effect on people.

Berenice had had a fever and swollen organs, but she was only one patient, and she returned to good health after two weeks. Her fever faded, and Dr. Chagas could barely see the parasite in her blood samples. Berenice was out of the acute stage of the infection and into the chronic one.

Then Dr. Chagas had the chance to autopsy the body of an infant who had been infected with *T. cruzi* and died. After carefully removing tissue samples from the baby's heart, Dr. Chagas shipped them to Dr. Gaspar Vianna, a pathologist at the Oswaldo Cruz Institute, who located the parasite in the tissue. Dr. Chagas carried out other autopsies and came to understand that the parasite leaves lesions on the wall of the heart. If a person lived in an area with kissing bugs and had heart problems, he realized, they most likely had the disease in its chronic form.

As much as he tried, Dr. Chagas could not prove that thousands of people in Brazil were suffering from the disease. He was nominated twice for the Nobel Prize but did not receive it and died in 1934.

In the 1940s, Dr. Salvador Mazza was able to find more than a thousand cases of the kissing bug disease in Argentina. He did it by screening patients with a particular combination of symptoms: fever, fatigue, and irregular heartbeats. Dr. Cecilio Romaña, who worked with him, figured out that if the parasite enters a person's eye by way of the conjunctival sac, the eyelid can swell and turn the color of violets, or a shade of pink. The swelling is distinct—a giant marble under the eyelid. This symptom, now called Romaña's sign, indicates the acute stage of the kissing bug disease. It can last more than a month before the person moves into the chronic stage.

How does a parasite end up in a person's eye?

After the kissing bug bites a person (or any mammal), it defecates. This is critical because the parasite is bundled in the insect's feces. A person can rub their arm or face where the kissing bug attacked and defecated, then touch their eyes with the same hand, effectively transferring the insect's feces and *T. cruzi*.

With this new information from Argentina, doctors all over South America, Central America, and Mexico looked for the kissing bug disease in rural areas where the triatomine insects make their home. By 1985, more than seventeen million people were thought to be infected with the parasite.

...

Berenice, the toddler, lived for decades with *T. cruzi*. When reporters tracked her down in the 1960s, she was in her early fifties. She had kept a doll and a medal that Dr. Chagas had given her and also this memory: the man with the long face had wanted to take her to Rio de Janeiro to become a scientist. He had apparently harbored a dream that the patient who had made it possible for the world to know about this parasitic disease would one day work in medical research. Her parents, however, did not let her go.

Berenice lived to be seventy-three years old. She died, apparently unharmed by the parasite, in 1981, the same year I turned six and stood in my family's living room with a nurse, translating for my auntie.

...

Tía Dora did not know this history of the disease, and I did not know it either when she was alive. We did not, in general, discuss her illness. Then again, maybe we didn't have the time. We were always fighting.

PELEAS

My first fight with Tía Dora occurred over love. It happened in 1981, after her initial surgery. She felt well enough to slip my baby sister, Liliana, into a summer dress and push her in the stroller down our block in Union City. My sister looked like baby Jesus with my auntie as the virgin mother. They were a minor sensation in the neighborhood. The Cubanas loved seeing them, and my sister, as a newborn, looked a lot like Tía Dora, with the same dainty lips and button nose. Both wore summer dresses as if cotton had been invented for their bodies.

No one mistook me for Tía Dora's child.

My eyes, round and long-lashed, did not belong to her, and my lips were too full, and also I was inclined, even at the age of six, toward hard corners. I stuffed Barbies into a toy car and sped them down hallways to see them crash. I played catch with the boys until a baseball smashed my eye and blood gushed from my nose. I insisted on crossing the street solita without holding anyone's hand. Everyone could see it in me, especially Tía Dora: I intended to swallow the world whole.

Back in the apartment, Tía snuggled with Liliana on her lap. My mother had covered the red sofa with plastic like every Latina family we knew in the early eighties in Jersey. I poked at the hard plastic and screamed at Tía Dora to stop paying attention to my sister, to play with me instead.

Tía giggled and turned to my mother. "¡Tiene celos!"

I cried that I was not jealous, and I don't know what I did after that. Maybe I threw the Barbie at the floor. Maybe I begged. All I know is that we never stopped fighting.

...

From Tía Dora's perspective, she did not demand much of me. She simply wanted me to be like my sister, who did not argue with her. Liliana agreed to everything over the years: the pigtails, the itchy school socks, the cereal bowl with too much milk. She knew how to go along to get along, and since we did not have other siblings and all our cousins were in Colombia and Cuba, my sister and I became a painful study in contrasts for my auntie.

To the same degree that my sister charmed her, I horrified Tía Dora. I did not want her combing my hair and I would not comb it when she told me to. I did not smile at her when I woke up in a foul mood. I joined adult conversations, scowling when I disagreed. I said what was on my mind and I didn't care what anyone thought. I behaved, in other words, like a boy.

When we moved a few miles north from the apartment in Union City to the house with the kitchen-garden, Tía Dora came with us. My parents worked in textile factories, and so it was Tía who poured orange juice for us, who walked us across the street to school— Liliana in first grade and me in sixth. One morning, Tía Dora explained, "When you hear your name called, you say, 'Señora?'"

"That's ridiculous," I said.

Why should I say "¿Señora?" the Spanish equivalent of "Ma'am?" when someone came looking for me? It made more sense to reply, "What do you want?" Tía Dora glared at me. When she was angry, her long chin looked pointier, and she drew it in as if I had offended that part of her face. It was like watching a silent movie. Her chin pulled in. Her forehead creased. Her eyes slowly moved toward the green apples on the kitchen wallpaper. She'd had enough of me. I was dismissed.

...

Some years, we had ridiculous arguments. Tía Dora wanted me to walk into the kitchen in the mornings, see her at the table, and greet her with a kiss on the cheek and a "Buenos días." Apparently, this was what all well-behaved teenagers did in Bogotá. It was what my sister did in Jersey. I was the only one having a problem with good manners.

"Buenos días," Tía called to me from the kitchen table.

I grunted and reached for the cereal box. She turned to my mother and declared, in Spanish, "La india is in a bad mood."

When a Colombian auntie calls you an Indian, it means you're behaving badly. Tía Dora gave me a long look, then pursed her lips and turned the conversation to monkeys. "Tiene el mico," she said, as if I weren't in the room. This was her go-to phrase: the Colombian equivalent of saying, "You have a monkey on your back." It drove me crazy: the constant commentary on my moods and movements, even my facial expressions.

Liliana knew to stay in our living room, focused on cartoons. Already she was afraid of me, afraid of how I stomped up and

51

down the stairs, of the way I had learned from my father to curse in Spanish. She was learning to be like my mother, una muñeca, and to stay out of the way.

Tía Dora rose from the kitchen table and called to my sister, "Liliana." My sister, her hair in pigtails the size of dark plums, sweetly replied, "Señora?"

...

For years, when friends complained to me about domineering mothers, I said nothing. My mother hemmed my school uniform skirts and cleaned the kitchen and mostly let me do anything I wanted. I wore bright red lipstick. I convinced Mami to pay a lady in the neighborhood to give me an at-home perm. I wore an off-the-shoulder T-shirt like Madonna and breezed past my mother's silent, pained face.

But the longer my friends lamented about mothers who tried to micromanage their lives, the more their complaints felt familiar. I thought about Tía Dora. I realized I had that mother too.

...

One topic we never argued about was the kissing bug disease. Tía Dora insisted on silence about it, and I agreed. She hid it from her new friends in Jersey, and when she received her teaching certification and landed a job teaching Spanish in an elementary school, she did not tell her coworkers. No matter how mad I was, I never snitched. It was her secret, and at the age of thirteen, I knew not to betray her. Besides, most days, she was fine. Flaca but fine.

I thought of the disease as solid and inarguable, like the peri-odic table that hung in the science classroom at my high school. Who debates helium? Nickel or cobalt? I accepted without ques-tion that each element has its structure, its name, its place on the table and on the planet. I felt the same about the kissing bug disease and Tía's body. It was a matter of fact.

And we also never argued about the man who proposed to marry her.

. . .

The man from Peru who wanted to marry Tía Dora wore ironed slacks and polo shirts. He had a luminous, indigenous face, and a thick set of glasses that made him look like a scholar. He and my auntie met in an English class, a year or two after her surgeries. Tía liked that he read the newspapers, and that when she called his name, he dutifully replied, "Señora?"

The other aunties and my mother whispered that he had been a radio announcer in Peru. In New Jersey, he worked at a printing factory, carting home bundles of discarded paper for typewriters. He gifted me the empty pages, and though his name was José, I think of him now as Tío Papeles, the Paper Uncle. I stacked the pages on my corrugated wood desk and waited for a story to write.

Tío Papeles was not like the other men in our family. He stayed away from beer and ate in moderation. He enunciated his words. He did not work every day of the week. He drove a Chevrolet. Because of Tío Papeles, we traveled by car to the supermarket, the shopping mall, and Bear Mountain State Park. Because of Tío Papeles and his Nikon camera, photographs document our childhoods: my sister and me with Tía Dora on the Palisades and at the Christmas tree at Rockefeller Center and at the park under the George Washington Bridge. Because of Tío Papeles, we had a father during the Reagan years when Papi worked long hours at the textile factory and chased after side jobs on his days off.

I was nine the summer Tío Papeles and Tía Dora took us to a lake in Jersey. Giant coolers dotted the grassy area and burgers sizzled on the grills. Shirtless, Tío Papeles looked like a god from the Inca Empire. I followed him into the lake filled with children and grown-ups bobbing in the water and tossing beach balls. Tío put his leg into the water so that his right thigh was at a ninety-degree angle. I climbed onto his leg and stood up, my right hand on his shoulder, the lake spreading before me like a massive blue sheet. My tío told me to dive. I hesitated. He said, "Aquí estoy. Brinca." His voice sounded so confident, and his shoulder firm like dry land, so trustworthy. I jumped.

My chin dipped into the cool water. Then my nose, my cheeks, my forehead, my chest, my belly, tumbled. I sank, untethered, and the silence startled me. The children's laughter vanished. My tío's voice, gone too. I reached out for something, anything, but finding nothing, I flailed my arms. Then, as if he truly were an Incan deity, Tío Papeles plunged his hands in and plucked me up and out of the lake. I loved it: the adrenaline, the rescue, the safety of his arms.

That summer, Tío Papeles taught me to float, to lean back and trust the water. "Open your eyes this time," he said, in Spanish, and I did, enough to see the wispy clouds shape-shifting in the blue sky.

...

That summer when I thought of Tío Papeles as an Inca god, he was actually already wed to a Puerto Rican woman for his green card. He wanted to marry Tía Dora, but first he had to wait for his divorce papers. So they put off the legal part of the wedding (the trip to city hall, the marriage license), but not the church ceremony. Tía bought the dress, and the church rented them the hall five days before Christmas in 1985.

We spent that fall submerged in fabric. My mother came home from the factory, and after dinner and washing the dishes, she sat on the bed late into the night, stitching sequins to the wedding dress. The fabric, cream and voluminous, stretched across the entire bed. A Victorian-style dress, with a high collar and long sleeves, it covered almost every inch of Tía's body and made her look heavier, healthier.

Tía Dora and Tío Papeles were a handsome couple. When they married that December, it felt to me that they had already lived a life together. They moved into his apartment and bought a television screen and watched movies together. On weekends, they hosted parties and drove my mother, my sister, and me to visit Colombian and Peruvian friends in Long Island and Queens. One year I won a prize in an essay contest, and the two of them arrived at our house smartly dressed and whisked us away to pick up the award.

Two years later, Tío Papeles did get divorced from the other woman, and he legally married Tía Dora, who was by then under an order of deportation. He swore in writing to the US federal government that he would take responsibility for her. And it worked. My auntie received permanent legal status.

Together, Tía Dora and Tío Papeles convinced my mother to buy me a set of the Encyclopaedia Britannica. I was in middle school and they were the first books I owned. My mother and I arranged them in a bookcase in my bedroom, then sat back to admire the golden foil of the letters on the spine of each volume. The encyclopedias felt to me like the epitome of the eighties, like Tía Dora's life with Tío Papeles: extravagant. Some days, the joy proved so keen that all I could do was thumb through a single volume to feel its silky pages in my hands.

...

I never consulted the encyclopedia about the kissing bug disease, and I wonder if it would have explained how *T. cruzi* favors the hollow organs of the human body. How the heart, for all the metaphorical language imposed on it, is a hollow organ. The encyclopedia did have exquisite pages depicting the human body, including the gastrointestinal system. The esophagus looked innocent on those pages: a curious ribbon the color of cream twirling in midair, a part of the body that would never betray a woman. But in 1992, when I was seventeen and Tía forty-one, her esophagus began to unravel.

At first, she couldn't swallow. It hurt when she tried, as if her throat had suddenly shrunk. She spent days vomiting, and when she tried to eat, she ran a fever. The details are hazy and the medical records lost from that year, but we know this much: she had esophageal surgery. The damage *T. cruzi* inflicts on the esophagus is similar to the large intestine—it eats away at the neurons necessary for making the organ move. In this way, *T. cruzi* can kill a person by starving them.

Tía survived the surgery and was bed-ridden for eight months. She praised the nurses in almost religious tones. "Con una delicadez," she said about how they touched her body with such attentiveness, such sweetness. Finally, permitted to eat, she began very slowly, cautiously picking up a spoonful of rice as if the grain might prove perilous.

...

The year I turned seventeen Tía Dora was probably not speaking to me. We both agreed, I think, that Bill Clinton should win the presidency that November, but she hated my boyfriend. It did not matter that he was like her: light-skinned, Colombian, an immigrant. All she could see was that he was flipping burgers at McDonald's. She, meanwhile, had gone through all the paperwork to have her college degree from La Salle University in Bogotá validated in the United States. She had taken college courses in New York for a year. She was certified to work as a substitute teacher, a bundle of ambition, and there I was: her US-born sobrina, proffering my love and my body to a boy she would not have considered in her own country. I thought she was a snob. She insisted she was right.

In generous moments now, I believe the hardest part of my relationship with Tía Dora sprang from a feud neither of us understood. Perhaps the reason was grounded in cultural differences or generational ones (she was a baby boomer immigrant, I was a Gen X American). But my sister adored her and so did our young cousins in Colombia. This makes me think that our differences existed beyond the hard fabric of time and place. I am sure that if we had been born in the same generation, or a hundred years earlier in the same country, we still would have been at odds. I would have been a suffragette on the lecture circuit in the United States, and she would have pulled in her chin and complained that I should be content with my teaching job.

...

A year after Tía had esophageal surgery, Tío Papeles fainted on the floor of the printing factory. The hot weather that July in 1993 made his coworkers think he'd had a heatstroke, and he was rushed to the emergency room. Everyone was confident that he'd be back to work in another day or two. But Tío Papeles had stomach cancer. Tío Papeles would shrink. Tío Papeles would die within the year.

His death felt like a blindness. When he was diagnosed, I was eighteen and in my first year of college. I pretended it wasn't happening. I did what my father had taught me to do: work until the days vanish. I kept my two part-time jobs and moved in with my Colombian boyfriend and avoided Tío Papeles. I did not believe he would actually die.

Tía Dora hated airplanes, but Tío Papeles wanted to die with his mother in Peru. So I imagine that when the plane took off, Tía Dora shut her eyes and braced herself. She probably gripped his hand, which by then had become so withered she could feel the bones and tendons. She prayed, invoking the Virgin Mother and the Holy Father, and she opened her eyes and there she was, in the clouds with the man she loved bound for his homeland.

A month later, Tío Papeles was dead, his ashes joined to water and land that had once belonged to the Inca Empire. Everyone—the women in my family, the women in our community—whispered the same observation for months: "Dora's the one who is sick, but he's the one who died."

. . .

In 2000, six years after Tío Papele's death, Tía Dora began vomiting and running a fever. It hurt when she swallowed. Her esophagus, that string of ribbon, was dilated again, was losing its shape in her body and refusing to let her eat.

That was the year of tubes: tubes in her nose, tubes to her stomach, tubes to get her nutrients. Every time we thought the medical world had saved her; we didn't realize it was only granting her time.

It was also the year I decided to come out to my family. While I was terrified of telling them that I was bisexual, I was twenty-five and overconfident about their love. I believed they would work it out somehow. My mother did. My father too. But not Tía Dora. She stopped speaking to me, and I retreated into silence and nurtured a fantasy: if Tío Papeles had lived, he would have forced Tía Dora to call me. He would have told her that to be homophobic is to be backward. That queer people have existed since the beginning of time. He would have taken Tía Dora to the Met and shown her ancient art, the provocative gaze of the men for each other. He was dead, however, and she was alive and we didn't speak for the next seven years.

Tía Dora had adjusted to life without my uncle and now she did the same with me. She spent two summers in Spain, working on her graduate degree in Spanish. She landed a full-time job in Jersey, teaching young children—Latinx, African American, Muslim American children—the days of the week in Spanish and the history of Cinco de Mayo. A local Spanish-language newspaper published her op-ed on the importance of learning Spanish. She bought a computer and a printer and crammed them into the bedroom she had once shared with Tío Papeles.

The silence between us broke when she thought I was dating a cisgender man again. She never said it this way, but I don't think she actually cared that I was bisexual. Identity was irrelevant. She cared about who I was dating—the behavior. In the photograph I sent home from my new apartment in California, she saw me with a handsome Chicano and asked my sister, "Is this a real man?"

After three decades, Liliana still knew to stay out of our arguments. "Look at the picture," she told Tía Dora.

The photograph showed a tall man with gorgeous black hair and generous eyebrows. It did not indicate that he identified as transgender. The image did not hint at the vial of testosterone or the scars where surgeons had removed his breasts. The photograph hid everything about him that was trans, everything about us that was queer, and Tía Dora started speaking to me again, and after so many years of silence, I did not argue with her. I had missed her.

Two years later, I found myself again interpreting between Tía and an English-only nurse except this time it was in an emergency room.

IT SOUNDS WORSE IN SPANISH

That night at Hoboken University Medical Center we had a room with a door and a curtain to yank around the gurney. The walls were the color of pale eggshells.

I was grateful for the door. I did not want my auntie hearing the yelps and cries of other people in the ER. Not tonight. For the first time in my life, I had been the one to bring my auntie to the hospital. Not a family friend, not a taxi, not a neighbor. Me. A torch had been passed. I lived across the country but was in town for a visit, and at thirty-five, I was finally old enough to take care of my auntie by myself.

The stiff edge of the chair pushed into the backs of my legs. I didn't take off my winter coat. On the gurney, Tía Dora lay on her left side, her hand tucked under her cheek. She was fifty-nine and looked like a shrunken fairy from a children's storybook. She refused to tell me how much she weighed, but the paperwork I received later stated eighty pounds. The bones in her wrists pressed against her thin skin. Her hair, honey brown and straight, had split ends, and she licked her cracked lips repeatedly. She was dehydrated. She had been vomiting for two days and had severe abdominal pains.

White coats came and went. They wanted blood. They wanted to hook her up to an IV. They wanted X-rays.

From the gurney, Tía Dora raised her bony right index finger and waved a "no" to the X-rays.

"¿Por qué no?" I asked.

She whispered in Spanish, "They'll get scared when they see the X-ray."

I didn't argue with her. In general, we did not argue in hospitals. We acted like reasonable women who got along, who agreed on politics, who braided each other's hair. If Norman Rockwell had painted Latina women for the cover of the *Saturday Evening Post*, he would have depicted me that night in the ER with my hair in a tight ponytail, my oval face strained in worry, my hands pulling a shawl over the hospital gown to cover Tía Dora's frail shoulders. Rockwell might have titled the piece *La Hija*.

Tía Dora had terrible pains in her lower belly. Finally a nurse arrived. He had thick fingers. He started to examine her, but Tía Dora's eyes flashed open in horror at his touch, and she screamed out in pain, her mouth a dark cavern. I stood there helpless and silent, holding her hand.

The doctors ordered IV fluids to counter the dehydration, and the next day, they sent her home.

...

Back in her apartment, Tía Dora told me about her trip to Colombia the year before. She had gone to see a doctor familiar with the kissing bug disease as her symptoms had worsened. She had lost a lot of weight. She knew that doctors in the United States rarely saw this disease. She was hoping this doctor could offer a new course of treatment. The physician followed protocols: a screening to check my auntie's body for antibodies to *T. cruzi*.

As she told me this, I sat at her dining table with a bowl of chicken soup. Tía Dora had tried to eat some broth, but it was too much for her. She stood from the table. She wore a heavy sweater layered over a blouse to try to hide how skinny she was, but that day nothing helped. She looked like a stick person a child might draw on a piece of paper, the clothing awkward boxes around her body.

What happened with the tests?

"He said I don't have Chagas," she told me.

"What?"

She didn't have the antibodies. "But then what do I have?"

The doctor didn't say. We wondered if we'd had the wrong diagnosis for decades, but later when I spoke to her physician in Jersey, Dr. Steven Goldstein, he couldn't imagine what else Tía Dora could have. She might have tested negative for the antibodies to *T. cruzi*, but she had all the clinical signs of the disease: her intestines unraveling, an esophagus that refused food.

Later, I learned that the parasite loves to hide in the human body. That negative test results can be a mistake. That the CDC requires several tests to confirm a positive diagnosis.

...

We didn't have enough time to look for answers. Two months later, Tía Dora was in the hospital for a scheduled procedure when her heart stopped. The medical team revived her, and when I arrived at the hospital from a cross-country flight, she was in the cardiac intensive care unit, on a ventilator. I grabbed her right hand and said, "Aquí estoy."

Her eyes widened, and she gripped my hand. Liliana stood at the foot of the bed near my mother, Auntie Biblia, and Radio Auntie, all of who were, by then, in their sixties and seventies. We prayed, but Tía Dora's heart stopped again. The medical team rushed in and barked at us to leave. They revived Tía, and when they yanked back the curtains, a nurse said, "If her heart stops again, she might not make it."

I nodded but didn't believe her. My auntie had been in and out of hospitals most of her life. Doctors had never known about the kissing bug disease, and they didn't know about it now. To me, she was not the kind of woman who died. She was a woman who lived close to death.

Back in the room, Tía Dora's eyes had stopped blinking. No one told us that she had slipped into a coma. The ventilator hissed and beeped. I asked a nurse, "Is it okay for her to have her eyes open like that?"

The nurse left the room and returned with gauze. Gently, her fingers pressed under my auntie's thin right eyebrow and coaxed the lid down. I looked away. When the nurse left, I saw she had covered each eye with gauze. Where Tía Dora's eyes should have been, now only two white wounds stared back at me.

It was after one in the morning. We sent Radio Auntie home in a taxi. The nurses' station glowed with its fluorescent overhead lights. The hospital rooms had grown silent, the curtains pulled open so nurses could keep an eye on the patients, all of whom were viejitos, their faces wrinkled from living full lives. My auntie, at fifty-nine, was probably the youngest patient in the cardiac ICU that night.

Liliana and I sat in hard chairs at the foot of Tía Dora's bed and listened to the ventilator. My sister was twenty-nine with a federal government job in Washington, DC, and soon policy makers would cite her research to encourage more states to grant college tuition waivers to foster youth. She had a plump face now, more our mother's daughter than Tía Dora's, and as the minutes passed, we started making plans for how we would take care of Tía when she recovered because we knew she would, as she had so many times before.

The vital signs monitor howled, and the physicians ran in again. Liliana stammered, "I'll get them," and she ran to the waiting room for my mother and Auntie Biblia. I waited and stared at the drawn curtains. Suddenly my sister was sprinting back around the nurses' station, almost skidding on the clean floor. My mother and Auntie Biblia trotted behind her, pocketbooks still dangling from their shoulders. We formed a circle outside Tía's room. Auntie Biblia implored God to help.

A doctor stepped out from the room, a woman with round brown eyes. She stared directly at me, and silently, she swung her head to the right.

I waited.

Her head only swung in the other direction.

I narrowed my eyes.

The doctor swung her head again.

Behind me, the women in my family burst into chaos. My sister sobbed. Auntie Biblia wailed. My mother cried a prayer.

The doctor told me, "Give them a few minutes and then you can go in."

My sister's shoulders trembled. My mother's feet tapped the floor anxiously. Auntie Biblia grabbed my arm. I thought: No. The doctor has made a mistake.

Inside the room, Tía Dora, free of all the machines, all the wires, even the ventilator, looked more like herself than she had in a long time. She appeared asleep on a table of pale marble, her hands clasped over her belly. The gauze had been removed, and her face was the one I had known for thirty years: the pale eyelids, the thin lips, the chin still pointing at me.

...

In the middle of the night, we shuffled out of the hospital and returned to Tía Dora's apartment where we tried to sleep but instead cried and finally, though it was not yet daybreak, Auntie Biblia declared the hour decent enough to start the necessary phone calls. From the sofa bed, I listened as she phoned her brother, Ernesto, in Colombia. "Dora se nos fue," she cried, but my uncle didn't understand. Dora had left? Where had she gone? Was she lost?

Numb, I took the phone receiver from my auntie and heard myself say, "Dora murió." She died. In Spanish, the words felt ancient. Dora murió. It sounded like I was talking about Catholic churches, black lace gloves, heavy ruanas. Dora murió. It sounded so much worse in Spanish.

CALL IT GRIEF

A few weeks after Tía Dora's death, my father had a massive stroke while waiting at a bus stop in Miami. Then the man I wanted to marry decided he wasn't sure he would ever walk down the aisle, and an editor I helped to hire pushed me out of a job I loved. I lost all sense of narrative structure in life, of "I feel *this* because *that* happened." Was I in shock about my auntie dying or Papi almost dying or me losing my job? Was I grieving the man I loved or Tía Dora?

The days took the shape of weeks, but the mourning lost all its edges and became a suffocating blanket. In Miami, where my parents had moved after my sister and I left home and the factories left Jersey for other places, the surgeon explained that my father would slowly recover the use of his right arm and leg and, later, his full vocabulary. The stroke had affected the part of his brain that connected words with objects, so in the rehab center, where he spent several weeks, Papi insisted one afternoon, "Give me the pen!" I dug one out of my bag and handed it to him. He barked, "What are you giving me this for?"

"You said you wanted a pen."

"Why would I want this? I don't want this. Give me the pen!"

My mother, patient as always, asked, "What do you want to do with the pen?"

"I'm going to change the channel!" he cried and slumped back in bed.

My mother handed him the remote control, and this happened several times with other objects: the fork, the slippers, the reading glasses. No matter how hard Papi tried, he could not correctly match his words to the intended object.

The same was happening to me. I could not point at a situation and call it grief. Every object I looked at—the plastic cups at the nurses' station, the folded bedsheets in the rehab center, the black flip-flops on my feet—every object could have been named grief.

I told myself not to be ridiculous. I was not grieving my dead auntie. I couldn't be—our relationship had been hard. I had nothing to mourn, and I did exactly what Tía Dora would have wanted me to do at that point, what she had done after Tío Papeles died: I threw myself into work. I finished a memoir and applied for grants. I left my apartment and friends in California, moved to South Florida, and started a master's program. I wrote a novel. I taught creative writing. And I started drafting a short story about the kissing bug disease.

...

When summer arrived in South Florida in 2013, three years after Tía Dora's death, I had managed my fear of bichos enough to read voraciously about kissing bugs. I learned that the baby insects are called nymphs, have five larval stages, and need to suck on blood to start molting. Although there are 140 species of these insects, only five are really responsible for transmitting *T. cruzi.* The faster a kissing bug defecates after biting, the more vulnerable the person might be since the parasite passes through the insect's feces. A friend in Miami cocked her head and joked, "It's like a crazy girlfriend. She breaks your heart, then shits on you."

It rained to extremes that summer. I scoured online science articles on kissing bugs, as my cat and I monitored the rainfall from the windowsill of our bedroom. One day, I clicked on a link and practically jumped from my chair when an image burst onto my screen of kissing bugs—dead and preserved and arranged in a line like foot soldiers. They reminded me of giant cockroaches, with wings and legs so long they looked like they could jump, which they can't, and their eyes—the insects have enormous eyes and petite heads. I shivered, then squinted at the photograph. Some of the kissing bugs had orange stripes at the edges of their backs, as if there were a god who had realized her mistake in making these six-legged creatures and at the last moment had thought to redeem them with pumpkin-striped skirts.

When it stopped raining, I opened the door to go for a walk and found a huge dead cockroach on the threshold, its rigid body flipped so the feet stabbed the air. I yelped and slammed the door shut. I told myself that it was not a kissing bug, only a cucaracha, and it was dead. I paced the kitchen, hyperventilating and remembering how, when I first looked for an apartment in Miami, one landlord had said, "They're palmetto bugs," as if I didn't know a cockroach when I saw one.

In the bedroom, my cat, Zami, napped on the windowsill. She did not kill rodents or roaches. A rescued Persian mix, she knew better than to associate with anything filthy enough to have six legs and antennae. She opened her eyes briefly to see me standing there, then stretched and curled into a tighter ball.

Finally, I gathered courage. The apartment had two doors to the street. I opened the second door in the living room slowly, saw the threshold free of horrors, and sneaked out of the apartment. Tía Dora would have done the same. If she were with me, she would have cried, "¡Asco!" about the dead roach and inched close behind me to tiptoe out. In the park near my apartment, the one with the gazebo, she would have slipped her arm into mine and walked with me as if she were a young royal on a stroll in the village square. I would have confessed: "I don't know why I am grieving you. You were awful to me, and yet here I am crying in public."

...

I convinced myself that my research into the kissing bug disease did not have much to do with Tía Dora. I had grown up in the shadow of a disease about which I knew little. Now I was reading that one study put the global cost of the kissing bug disease as higher than cervical cancer in terms of health care expenses and years of life lost. What else didn't I know?

The more I read, the more I began to appreciate the places where disease and politics intersect. Pathogens don't care about bank accounts, national boundaries, or tax returns, and yet government policies about race, class, and citizenship determine who gets to see a doctor and who gets treatment—in the simplest and scariest terms, who gets to live or die. If Tía Dora had arrived in the United States today rather than in 1980, she would have had to wait five years and needed a green card to qualify for Medicaid in some states. In all likelihood, the only reason the health insurance from her teaching job covered her later surgeries and hospitalizations was that the insurance agents did not know Tía Dora had a preexisting condition. It was hard to imagine any of them had heard of the kissing bug disease.

Tía Dora was actually the only woman in our family who had health insurance. My mother and Auntie Biblia worked in textile factories. Radio Auntie was a home health aide in Manhattan. When the summer arrived, my mother and tías took a public bus in Jersey to a feria de salud in West New York. The health fairs were held in church parking lots under bright blue canopies. Or in public parks. The white coats spoke Spanish and arranged the tables so that it was clear where my mother and Auntie Biblia and Radio Auntie were to go for blood pressure, azucar, and cholesterol screenings. Sometimes a woman offered a cooking lesson: how to make a fruit salad, how to stuff a red bell pepper. Mami snacked on crackers and watched, delighted at the woman's ease with the knife and the cutting board. Volunteers handed out plastic bags with information about how to keep bad cholesterol down.

The other way women in our immigrant neighborhood received health care was by word of mouth. That was how my mother learned that a clinic in Harlem gave women annual mammograms without charge, and she went every year until she reached the age to qualify for Medicare.

I did not have health insurance growing up. I did not have health insurance when I was eighteen and tripped in front of a store while running. My face smashed into the uneven asphalt, the skin on my chin tearing so that blood poured down my neck and my body shook, and my boyfriend at the time winced when he saw my face: a triangle of flesh exposed on my chin. Back home in our kitchen, my mother didn't know what to say. Who had the money for stitches? For an emergency room trip? I wasn't dying.

When I read articles labeling the kissing bug disease a "disease of poverty" and noting that about three hundred thousand people in the United States were infected, I wondered: Who are these families? Where are their stories? And also: are these families like mine? Before the Affordable Care Act passed in 2010, the least likely group to be insured were Latinas and Latinos, but having the kissing bug disease requires constant contact with doctors.

It turned out that Tía Dora was also part of a migratory shift when it came to the kissing bug disease. Growing economic inequities in South America and the brutal civil wars in Central America had pushed people to move to Spain, Italy, Japan, the United States, and many other countries. These were people who, like Tía Dora, had contracted *T. cruzi* from kissing bugs in their home countries. Now these women and men were waking up in European and American and Asian cities with hearts that felt too big for their chests, and doctors strained to understand why people in their forties had heart failure for no apparent reason.

...

Almost a year after I started reading about kissing bugs, Auntie Biblia phoned me to say she was making her annual trip to

Colombia for the anniversary of Tía Dora's death. A mass had been arranged in Bogotá.

"I want to go with you," I declared.

I did not tell Auntie Biblia about a professor I wanted to see in Bogotá. Felipe Guhl had an office at the most elite university in Colombia, and I had been tracking his work in scientific journals for months. While I was only beginning to learn details about the kissing bug disease, I had worked as a journalist for more than a decade. I knew people would talk to me, so I emailed the professor with links to articles I had published, described myself as a freelance reporter, and asked for an interview. It helped that he was very kind and that I had written for the *New York Times* in my twenties. He emailed back that, yes, he would meet with me at his office.

IN SEARCH OF
THE KISSING BUG

INSECTARIO

The day of my interview, the sky in Bogotá clouded early and stayed that way. I skipped the pink shawl and packed my black rain jacket. I was so nervous about my Spanish-speaking skills that I didn't look up as I walked across the campus of the University of Los Andes, which a relative of mine had referred to as the Harvard of Colombia. I moved forward, the campus map in hand, the security guard's directions on repeat in my mind. A minute later, I looked up.

The campus was tucked at the base of the mountain. Overhead, a sheet of brilliant green measuring more than ten thousand feet careened toward the sky. I turned around. I had climbed far enough that at my feet lay Bogotá with its skyscrapers and rapid bus system, its bundles of trees and the flat rooftops of bookshops and bakeries.

Later, I realized I was romanticizing the side of a mountain and the manicured grounds of an elite institution, but in that moment I did experience awe. This was a city whose geography did not permit erasure. I remembered my abuela, my mother's mother, who had a wide, wrinkled face, and how every time I looked at her I saw the mountain behind her. They became a single entity: my abuela-mountain. The days I spent with her began and ended with her wide skirts, the sensation in my toes of how tiny I was and how I was held by this woman, this mountain, this woman-mountain.

Three students strolled past me in sweaters. A fourth hurried. More of them sat on the green in tight knots of three and four, complaining about schedules and phone calls they had not received and people they knew. The building waited for me up ahead: the Center for Research in Microbiology and Tropical Parasitology.

...

I had not expected to find a mask of the Laughing Buddha in the professor's office, but there he was on the wall—past the jam-packed bookshelves, the tangle of conference badges hanging from a doorknob, and the L-shaped desk with its a wide-screen MacBook. The Laughing Buddha shared the space with a few masks that appeared African and Indonesian in origin. The professor had actually collected two hundred masks from more than thirty countries.

Professor Felipe Guhl reminded me of my tíos: salt-and-pepper hair, warm eyes, heavy at the waist, and smartly dressed in a wool sweater. A biologist, he had started studying the kissing bug disease in the seventies. Over the decades, he had, along with colleagues, mapped the places where fifteen species of kissing bugs make their homes in Colombia. He had found that houses in close proximity to the booming palm oil industry were particularly vulnerable to kissing bugs (the female insects stick their eggs to the palm leaves).

When Andean countries teamed up in the nineties to battle the kissing bug, he had been at the helm of the effort, and when we met in his office, he was at work with colleagues in several countries on the first double-blind study of the drug benznidazole, which can often cure people when they initially contract *T. cruzi*. The study focused on the drug's effect on people after that acute stage, when the parasite can lie dormant in the body for decades.

Professor Guhl leaned back in his office chair and reminded me that the kissing bug disease is a zoonotic disease—it jumps from wildlife to humans, like Lyme disease and the West Nile virus. More than 60 percent of emerging infectious diseases worldwide are zoonotic. And for that reason, the kissing bug disease cannot be wiped out. "To eradicate it would mean that you'd have to end all wildlife, right? And that is impossible," he said.

Although only five kissing bug species are considered dangerous in Latin America for their ability to transmit *T. cruzi*, there are more than a hundred species that could do the work, and this is another reason the disease is impossible to eradicate. "It's like a baseball game," Professor Guhl said. If pesticides eliminate one species of these insects, "there are other players on the bench." Some kissing bugs are seen only in the wild, he said, while others have become so habituated to living with people over time that they are usually only found in rural homes. I remembered that in the science literature, these are called "domestic" kissing bugs.

I must have looked crestfallen because Professor Guhl said, "You have to be clear about one point: it's one thing that a person is infected, and it's another thing that the person is sick."

Most people infected with *T. cruzi* do not get sick. They carry on with normal lives and die of other causes. But about 20 to

30 percent of those infected end up with cardiac problems, and fewer, like Tía Dora, with gastrointestinal issues. Only a small percentage of those who are sick actually die from the disease.

"Why and who develops symptoms is still a big question," Professor Guhl said, adding, "The parasite is very successful. It gets into the cells of the heart tissue. It stays there some time; then the intracellular forms get out and invade other new cells. But again all that depends on a lot of factors about which we still have a very big question mark."

Professor Guhl was eager to tell me that *T. cruzi* is not a single entity. There are actually six genetic groups, and, he explained, "each one of those trypanosomes has a distinct biological behavior."

Six types of this parasite?

"The frequency of *Trypanosoma cruzi* I is much greater" here in Colombia, he said. "So the pathology is also distinct." This parasite type causes heart damage, while another type, called *T. cruzi* II, is more likely to affect a person's gastrointestinal system.

I began to wonder if maybe my auntie didn't have this disease. Maybe she had something that looked like the kissing bug disease. Tía Dora's medical record was beginning to feel like that of Charles Darwin: sick her whole life and no one had a definitive answer.

Glancing at the clock, I realized I needed to ask Professor Guhl about the mummies.

...

The story of the kissing bug disease actually starts in one of the driest places on earth: the Atacama Desert. NASA compares this desert to the surface of Mars—it's hard to imagine life growing there given the rocky landscape, extreme temperatures, and ferocious winds dumping salt that never washes away. Straddling Chile and Peru, the desert spans more than six hundred miles and has no light pollution.

Atacama is where astronomers went to look for the ashes of stars that exploded after the Big Bang. It's where scientists traveled with a telescope to get the first picture of a black hole. Atacama is also the place where military men tossed the bodies of murdered activists during Chile's brutal dictatorship in the seventies and eighties. The desert held the bodies until the dictatorship ended and old women arrived, with small shovels, searching the desert for their sons and husbands, daughters and sisters.

At Atacama, Professor Guhl and an international team of researchers found mummies, one dating back nine thousand years, riddled with *T. cruzi.* In other words, the kissing bug disease existed in South America before Christopher Columbus arrived in the Carribbean. Testing close to three hundred mummies, Professor Guhl and his colleagues found that about 41 percent of them were infected with *T. cruzi.*

The parasite is only found in the Americas, where evidence of humans dates back fifteen thousand years. According to Professor Guhl, the mummies suggest that the parasite's "contact with humans in evolutionary terms is very recent." For the parasite, he added, "Humans are new. The parasite is trying to get the best deal, but it kills people, which, for him as a parasite, is not convenient."

I nodded. It was the first time I had heard someone talk about the parasite's point of view. It was the first time I had considered that a parasite had a point of view and a desire: it, too, wanted to stay alive.

...

Professor Guhl and I talked for an hour in his office, maybe longer. I could feel Tía Dora at my back, so I kept thanking him before asking another question. He teased that I should get out into the country and see the kissing bugs for myself. I wasn't quite sure how to tell an expert on triatomine insects that I thought anything with six legs was gross. I actually couldn't think of a word in Spanish for gross, or at least not one that I could use in a professional context.

Professor Guhl told me he had a colony of kissing bugs on campus for research purposes. I considered the opportunity. I was never going to travel into the wild to trap any insect. "Can I see the colony?" I asked.

Of course, he said, and arranged for one of his graduate students to give me a tour.

...

In Spanish, the room at the University of Los Andes that houses Professor Guhl's kissing bugs is called an insectario. From the outside, it looked like an ordinary room on campus with a locked door. I carried my notebook and swallowed my fear. A graduate student, taller than me and lanky, came with the keys.

It was a mild day in Bogotá, around sixty-four degrees Fahrenheit, but when the student pushed open the door to the bug room, it could have been summertime in North Carolina right after dusk. That is, the room was dimly lit and warm. Immediately, the student shut the door behind us, explaining that the room was temperature-controlled. I knew from reading articles that kissing bugs like the temperature to be between sixty-eight and eighty-six degrees Fahrenheit. In that temperature range, they'll feed about once a week. If it gets warmer, they'll want to bite a person, or any mammal or bird—what's called the host—more often. The lights had to be this dim too. Kissing bugs hate sunlight. They are nighttime feeders, and while other assassin bugs have curved proboscises, the kissing bug has a straight one, a needle-mouth it draws out to feed.

The room had three long wooden shelves filled with glass jars. Someone had folded black filter paper and stuffed it into each jar, then covered the tops with cheesecloth. The graduate student picked up a jar, and at first, I couldn't see anything inside. The student twirled the jar. The filter paper moved slightly, and a kissing bug poked its head out between the folds. To my surprise, it didn't look like a cockroach but rather something more substantial, perhaps a cross between a cucaracha and a beetle. I strained to see the colorful markings on its abdomen, but in the dark I could not see any distinguishing detail, just a six-legged bicho.

The kissing bug began crawling along the filter paper toward the lid of the jar. I froze, the notebook in my hands a necessary anchor as I stood, watching its six legs, its splayed antennae, its terrible four eyes. The first pair, located on the sides of the head, are the compound eyes insects usually have. Behind this set are another pair that can scan large areas.

A second kissing bug appeared between the folds of the filter paper, then another. They all climbed methodically, patiently. I stepped back. The graduate student turned the jar so I could see more kissing bugs hiding, their wings carefully tucked on their backs. Some were *Rhodnius prolixus*, less than an inch long. Some were nymphs but that didn't make them any less lethal—nymphs, too, can transmit the parasite for the kissing bug disease.

"What's at the bottom of the jar?" I asked.

The grad student peered closely. "The ones that died."

Every jar was a neighborhood of kissing bugs, and the bottom constituted an entomological cemetery littered with wing fragments and carcasses.

The room had been designed to please the kissing bugs: the dusky lighting, the warm air, the folds of paper in which they could hide. I began to appreciate that kissing bugs are homebodies. They make their homes near their supper, whether that's a human or an opossum or a German shepherd.

I knew from reading science articles that kissing bugs are not born with *T. cruzi* in their guts, but pick up the parasite when feeding on an infected host. It occurred to me that kissing bugs are innocent. They can transmit *T. cruzi*, yes, but they can also feed on a person or a family dog or a wild mammal, acquiring the parasite in the process. Kissing bugs are also the only insects known to transmit *T. cruzi* to people. Bedbugs can harbor the parasite, and in the laboratory, they have been shown to pass it along to mice, but scientists have not been able to explain why they don't do the same with humans.

The kissing bugs in the jar looked like they were walking with purpose. The graduate student smiled at me weakly. "They think we're going to feed them," he said. Their dinner? Chicken blood.

The graduate student had a kind, round face. "Are you scared of them?" I asked.

"I'm scared of *Panstrongylus geniculatus.*"

"Why?"

"It's long. It's like the length of my finger." He scanned the shelves as he said, "I'll show you one."

I wanted to tell him that it was fine, that I didn't need to see it, that I believed him. I was looking at his fingers to see if they were longer than mine when he said, "Here's one."

The jar looked a bit wider. He lifted it more carefully than he had the first jar, as if this giant kissing bug had already ripped the cheesecloth and was waiting for this moment to take flight from the jar and stab us with its needle-mouth.

The insect was longer, probably more than an inch. I couldn't make out any markings on its body. It hovered on the filter paper close to the bottom of the jar and looked half-asleep. I waited for it to move, to scuttle up the filter paper, to hunt for its supper, but the bug did not stir. I wondered if it was still satiated from its last blood meal.

...

Professor Guhl told me that battling the kissing bug means constant vigilance. A one-time fumigation of a rural house is not enough. In 1995, when forty-two scientists and researchers from fifteen countries gathered in Ecuador to discuss the insects and the disease, Guhl reported one of their conclusions: rural housing conditions have to be improved so kissing bugs don't have easy access to people.

Still, South America was winning the war against the kissing bug disease. According to the World Health Organization, the number of people infected had been steadily decreasing. In the nineties, between sixteen and eighteen million people were thought to have the kissing bug disease in Latin America, but today fewer than six million are infected. Maybe the decrease in infections was due to migration. People in Latin America, like those in the rural areas of the United States, were increasingly moving to the cities and away from the insects. Maybe it was due to a series of government initiatives that had begun in South America in the nineties and had raised awareness of the kissing bug disease and provided funds for fumigations. Maybe it was due to Doctors Without Borders and other nongovernmental organizations that had spent years in the region working with health ministers and local health care providers to make it possible for people to be tested for the disease and for children to be treated (children, for reasons doctors do not fully understand, can often be cured of the kissing bug disease even after the acute phase though the same isn't true for adults). Maybe Latin America was winning the war against the disease because the international health community had, at the start of the twenty-first century, begun paying attention to neglected tropical diseases in general. Experts convened conferences; declarations were issued. A list of neglected diseases was created. The list included the kissing bug disease as well as rabies, sleeping sickness, river blindness, leprosy, and leishmaniasis.

...

When I left the insectario, I did not think of staying in South America to write about the kissing bug disease. I was raised by an immigrant family in the United States, and the story I knew best was the one of migration, of negotiation, of borders that are imagined and frequently in flux. At the time of my visit to Bogotá in 2014, more child migrants were arriving at the US-Mexico border. Phil Gingrey, a congressman from Georgia, wrote to the CDC that summer, asking officials to "assess the public risk" the children posed with respect to diseases and to "provide guidelines to the public about how to protect themselves from potential infection." He told an NBC reporter that Border Patrol agents were worried about Ebola, tuberculosis, and the kissing bug disease. In the town of Murrieta, an hour north of San Diego, Americans turned away buses filled with migrant children. One picture taken by a Fox News photographer showed a woman with pale skin wearing hot pink shorts, holding a sign that read: "Save our children from diseases."

I stared at that three-letter word, the possessive pronoun "our" as in our children, our health, our country. The historian Alan M. Kraut calls it "medicalized nativism," when immigrants are linked to a disease and stigmatized. It worried me that this could happen with the kissing bug disease even though most people only become infected from direct contact with the insects. It would be like blaming people from Connecticut for Lyme disease. But the kissing bug disease is mostly found among immigrants from Latin America. That could make a difference.

There was another reason to return to the United States: the kissing bugs themselves. The insects are native to this country.

Historically, they have been found in warm spots like Texas, Arizona, California, and Louisiana. I began to wonder about the history of the disease in the United States, and then I learned about the medical experiment carried out in Texas on a young Black man.

AUSTIN STATE HOSPITAL

In the medical sketch, the young Black man has a shaved head and a clear face. He is twenty-four years old, almost six feet tall, and his left eye is closed, the lid swollen. His right eye stares at the artist.

I imagine that this young Black man is defiant, that he knows a part of his face is being documented, that he has something to say about it. Other times, I look at his eyes and can only consider the reality of his Black body, of what the white male doctor in South Texas did to his body, and then I believe that the young man in the sketch is thinking only of his left eye. He wants the swelling gone. He wants the fever to end too and his armpit not to bulge like a water balloon. He wants his body back intact.

It is the only image I find of him.

...

The sketch was included in a 1943 medical journal article titled "Infectivity of the Texas Strain of *Trypanosoma cruzi* to Man," and it was published by the *American Journal of Tropical Medicine and Hygiene*. When my university library sent me the article, I had not expected it to come with an image of a young Black man's face, but it did, and I spent hours, then days, then weeks, looking for his name. I turned up nothing. But the article's acknowledgments and a review of the author's archived correspondence revealed that the young Black man, in all likelihood, had been a patient at the first hospital in Texas for the mentally ill: the Texas State Lunatic Asylum.

The young Black man may have ended up in the asylum for any number of reasons. Since the institution's opening in 1861, people had been committed for drinking too much or being promiscuous or writing bad checks. By the late 1930s, about 70 percent of the patients were diagnosed either with schizophrenia or what is now known as bipolar disorder. The asylum's name was changed to Austin State Hospital, and by 1940, it had close to three thousand patients, housing Black patients in one ward and whites in another, and also separating them by gender. Distinct kitchens provided meals for white and Black patients. "Even the filing system was segregated," a social worker reported decades later. When the hospital first opened, Black patients slept in the basement.

One day in the winter of 1940, the young Black man from the medical sketch most likely joined a line of other Black men for breakfast. He wasn't the only patient in his twenties. There would have been others his age, as well as men in their fifties and older, all of them in Black pants and button-down shirts, the bowls in their hands wide enough for a cup of rice. Most likely the young Black man did not know what would be done to him that day. It was simply another Thursday morning in December. Perhaps he ate quickly while thinking of Christmas and the long stretch between what he wanted to buy for his family and what he could afford. He might have been a father, but I thought of him in relation to younger siblings: a sister he doted on, a brother he teased. The Second World War raged that winter. Maybe he overheard hospital workers talking about the Germans bombing London, first during daylight hours and then at night. Maybe he thought about the draft. It was new. Maybe he wanted to serve.

In Alabama, the Tuskegee syphilis study was underway that December. Federal public health officials were lying to Black men and their families, telling them that they were receiving treatments for "bad blood," as syphilis was called then, when in reality doctors were not treating them at all and were, instead, monitoring them for how the disease progresses in the Black body untreated.

At Austin State Hospital, the young Black man was taken to see a researcher who worked for the US Public Health Service, the same agency conducting the Tuskegee syphilis study. The researcher, Ardzroony Packchanian, had been asked to come to Texas to see what he could find about the kissing bug disease.

...

Packchanian was born in Armenia at the start of the twentieth century, so when he landed in New York City in 1921, he was still a young man. He may have considered himself lucky. He had not lost his life in the 1915 genocide that killed more than a million Armenians in the Ottoman Empire. He also arrived in the United States when the door was still open to immigrants. A few years later, Congress passed annual quotas on immigration limiting the entry of Armenians to a mere one hundred people (the quota for Germans numbered at more than twenty-five thousand). Packchanian's arrival in the United States then was marked by those bitter bookends: genocide and xenophobia.

Like so many immigrants then and now, he seems to have slipped into the racial category of whiteness with all its demands and benefits. He enrolled at the City College of New York, then studied at Columbia and Yale until he landed at the University of Michigan. He completed his doctoral work on sleeping sickness in animals.

By 1940, Packchanian had shifted his focus to the kissing bug disease and shown that a species of kissing bugs native to Texas could carry *T. cruzi* and transmit the parasite to mice, guinea pigs, and rhesus monkeys. News of his research had appeared in the *New York Times*. Now Packchanian wanted to know if humans could also contract the parasite from these local kissing bugs and develop symptoms.

...

Maybe the young Black man looked at Packchanian suspiciously. Maybe he wondered why the researcher was listening to his heart and noting that there was no sign of an irregular heartbeat. Maybe he kept an eye on the researcher's white hands.

Packchanian had collected kissing bugs of the species *Triatoma heidemanni* (now classified as *T. lecticularia*) from a town more than two hours south of Austin. In his makeshift laboratory, he crushed one of the kissing bugs. The insect's needle-mouth, its translucent wings, its abdomen and six legs—all were pulverized. Packchanian knew that an infected kissing bug in South America could transmit *T. cruzi* to humans. He knew, too, that at its worst the parasite could devour the human heart.

Packchanian pulled up the young Black man's left eyelid and forced part of the crushed insect into his eye. Less than an hour later, he also infected three mice and two guinea pigs.

Almost two weeks later, right before Christmas, the doctor could not find any sign of the parasite in blood samples taken from the young Black man, but the twenty-four-year-old began running a fever. The lymph nodes in his armpits ballooned. His left eye, suddenly bloodshot, pained him. He developed pink eye. His left eyelid swelled shut.

Forty-eight hours later, the swelling of his eyelid vanished. The fever persisted for another two weeks. And the parasite? Shortly after Christmas, it could be seen under the microscope vibrating in a droplet of the young man's blood.

...

It's hard to imagine that Packchanian explained the disease and the experiment to the young Black man. Harder still to imagine that the twenty-four-year old, perhaps diagnosed with schizophrenia, perhaps suffering from depression, perhaps guilty of nothing except being Black and male in South Texas, would have agreed to offer his body to science.

...

Six weeks later, in the middle of January, Packchanian placed several kissing bugs in a container covered with a cheesecloth lid.

These were healthy insects. He had reared them in the laboratory and monitored their blood feedings. Since a kissing bug has to feed on an infected host to catch *T. cruzi*, Packchanian must have felt confident. These kissing bugs, all of them nymphs, were free of the pathogen.

He strapped the container filled with the nymphs to the young Black man's forearm, and the insects raced toward his flesh and stuck their needle-mouths through the cheesecloth and into his skin, sucking up his blood.

When Packchanian dissected the insects and searched, he found the parasite. He repeated this test a week later and got the same results. It confirmed that he had infected the young Black man with *T. cruzi* from kissing bugs native to the United States.

The lymph nodes in the young man's armpits remained swollen for months.

. . .

While researching, I thought about Tía Dora and how she had been surrounded all her life by her sisters and me and my sister, and I wondered about the women who had loved this young Black man. His mother, maybe an auntie or a sister. Did they visit him for Christmas and worry about his fever? Did they bring him gifts? A new pair of socks? A hand-knitted cap for his shaved head?

. . .

In 1941, a year after he infected the young Black man, Packchanian could not find the parasite in the man's bloodstream. Almost two years later, the doctor declared him free of the parasite and also the disease.

It is difficult to find *T. cruzi* in the bloodstream once a person is in the chronic stage of the disease. The search has to focus on antibodies. In the 1940s, though, such antibody tests did not exist for the kissing bug disease. Maybe the young man lived unaffected by the parasite. Or maybe the parasite had found its way into his heart.

...

Packchanian went on to enjoy a long career as a professor at the University of Texas Medical Branch in Galveston. He had professional contacts with physicians from Argentina and Brazil who devoted their lives to the kissing bug disease, men like Salvador Mazza and Emmanuel Dias. And he spent a decade looking for people who had contracted the kissing bug disease in Texas, but he failed, it seems, to find a single one.

At first, I thought Packchanian had experimented on one patient. Then, after a librarian emailed me his medical correspondence, I found a letter from Garland G. Zedler, a doctor who had worked at Austin State Hospital that winter in 1940. He wanted to know what had come of Packchanian's experiments on hospital patients. Packchanian replied that he had not kept track of those cases, but, he wrote: "I am enclosing here a reprint describing one of the patients." The reprint was not included, but the phrase "one of the patients" jolted me. The young Black man had not been the only one.

In his published article, Packchanian thanked several people. He thanked the state's health department for the use of their labs and the superintendent of Austin State Hospital, Dr. C. H. Standifer, and also Dr. Zedler for "valuable clinical assistance in this case." *The American Journal of Tropical Medicine and Hygiene* published his article without comment.

PHARMA BRO

A year after my trip to Colombia, I obsessively dug into more historical texts about the kissing bug disease in the United States. I also interviewed experts, including cardiologists and an epidemiologist, and I published a piece online with *The Atlantic* about the disease. I wasn't the only one at work. My sister had moved to Virginia where the Latinx population had doubled between 2000 and 2010. She teamed up with advocates to convince the state legislature to pass a bill designating April 14 as Virgnia's "Chagas Disease Awareness Day." It was the date Dr. Carlos Chagas had first identified the parasite in the toddler Berenice.

I landed in Ohio for a teaching job, renting an apartment in a Cincinnati neighborhood lit by gas-fueled lamps, and often late into the evenings, I read the news online, which is how I first learned about the pharmaceutical executive Martin Shkreli. Newspapers had nicknamed him "the most hated man in America," and Donald Trump, then the leading Republican presidential candidate, had commented that the young man "looks like a spoiled brat."

In the fall of 2015, Shkreli's company hiked the price on the drug Daraprim from $13.50 to $750 a pill. Doctors prescribed this drug for toxoplasmosis, a parasitic disease I knew as the "cat litter disease." Although I had never been pregnant, I often noticed the labels on litter boxes warning pregnant women about handling cat litter on account of a parasite that cats can shed in their feces. Usually a person's immune system effectively battles this one-celled parasite, but it can turn fatal in babies or HIV-positive patients with weakened immune systems. Like the kissing bug disease, toxoplasmosis is linked to poverty and communities of color. Immigrants, Black Americans, and those with low incomes are more likely to have the disease. The drug Daraprim can save lives, but Shkreli's new pricing was putting it out of reach.

Everyone, it seemed, expected Shkreli to apologize and lower the drug price. He did not. He went on Bloomberg Television and defended the price increase. He showed up at the Forbes Healthcare Summit, and when asked what he would have done differently, he said, "I would have raised prices higher." He then spent $2 million on the only existing copy of a Wu-Tang Clan album and said he would play the album for a particular female singer in exchange for oral sex. On social media and in news accounts, Shkreli became known as the "pharma bro."

Shkreli was not the only executive guilty of raising drug prices by horrifying amounts. That same year, executives from Valeant Pharmaceuticals (now Bausch Health Companies) jacked the prices on the heart drugs Isuprel and Nitropress by 525 percent and 212 percent respectively, and Rodelis Therapeutics increased the price of a tuberculosis medication from $500 for thirty pills to more than $10,800 (the latter company reversed course when the news became public). A year later, the pharmaceutical company Mylan notoriously hiked the price on the EpiPen from $100 to more than $600 for two doses.

I suspected the reason Martin Shkreli bothered me and a good number of other people was that his price increase, and his arrogance, underscored a political reality: as Americans, we have choices about whom we take care of when it comes to health care and drug prices, but the ways to exercise these choices—by voting the right candidates into office and making demands of our elected officials—often feel intangible. Rather than organize for political change, it is easier to hate a young man who twirls a lock of brown hair on his forehead and makes vile sexual statements— a man who, in the summer of 2015, at the age of thirty-two, could with his words alone generate millions of dollars from investors and stop people from getting necessary, lifesaving drugs.

Martin Shkreli did not lower the price on the drug Daraprim, and a few months later, he came after benznidazole—a drug used to battle the kissing bug disease.

...

The World Health Organization considers benznidazole an "essential medicine," a treatment critical for global public health. The drug can often eradicate the parasite when a person first contracts it, and it can also do this, after the acute stage, for infected newborns, children, and teenagers. Studies have also found that women treated with benznidazole before pregnancy are less likely to pass the parasite to their children in utero.

Most people who have the kissing bug disease are in the chronic stage—many have been living with it for decades. Benznidazole, which interferes with the parasite's protein synthesis, reduces the parasite load in a person's body, and this might explain why an observational study in Argentina suggested that the drug helps people who are infected with the parasite but have not yet developed heart failure. The study that Professor Guhl had been working on—the first double-blind study of benznidazole and one that involved multiple countries—revealed that once the parasite has infiltrated a person's heart and begun to cause damage—and this can happen decades after the infection—the drug does not save the heart.

In 2015, benznidazole was not approved by the US Food and Drug Administration (FDA) so a person could only receive the drug by way of the CDC under certain protocols, and few people did. One study led by a clinical fellow from Harvard Medical School found that only 422 patients in the United States got the medication between 2007 and 2013, though an estimated three hundred thousand people here have the disease. It wasn't that the CDC denied a high number of requests. Most of these people didn't know they were infected. They were not sick nor were they screened. Tía Dora never took benznidazole. When she was alive, we didn't know it existed.

After raising the price on Daraprim and buying the Wu-Tang Clan album, Martin Shkreli bragged to investors that his company would convince the FDA to approve benznidazole in the United States. He boasted that this would generate millions of dollars in profit because the federal government had a financial incentive in place for pharmaceutical companies to bring drugs to the market for certain rare or "orphan" diseases. In filings with the Securities and Exchange Commission, Shkreli's company said it would price benznidazole similarly to medications for hepatitis C, which ran close to $100,000 for a course of treatment.

In South America, the cost of treatment with benznidazole was between $50 and $100. The CDC, when it sent the drug to physicians in the United States, charged nothing. It also didn't charge for another drug, nifurtimox, that was also used to treat people with the kissing bug disease. This drug was often not as well tolerated as benznidazole but the pharmaceutical Bayer had been donating the drug to the World Health Organization since 2002.

...

I have to guess that Martin Shkreli did not like the article I wrote about him for *The Atlantic*, in which I pointed out the racial impact of what he was proposing to do. He wanted to price a drug at close to $100,000 for a disease that mostly afflicts poor Latinx immigrants in the United States. He tweeted a single word at me after the article was posted: "Really?"

Part of me wanted to call him out on social media. Part of me realized that it was an opportunity for an interview. A Twitter exchange would be an imperfect interview, but my calls to Shkreli's company had not been returned. "Why up the price?" I asked him over Twitter, and he tweeted back: "Not FDA approved." I pointed out that he did not have to hike the price. He wrote back a painful and simple answer: "There is not a current price in the US for benznidazole." So he could set one.

Investors gave his company $8 million in the hopes of getting FDA approval for benznidazole.

The morning after Shkreli and I exchanged tweets, the FBI arrested him in his Manhattan apartment on charges of securities fraud. *Harper's* documented how Shkreli's notoriety made for difficult jury selection at his trial. One juror had a mother, grandmother, and brother with lifelong health issues that required access to medications, and the juror didn't think it would be possible to remain unbiased. Another juror, speaking of Shkreli, said, "I think he's a greedy little man," and a third juror said, "He kind of looks like a dick." More than two hundred people were excused from jury duty.

Shkreli's arrest did not stop his pharmaceutical company. It got a new president and later a new name, and the new president declared that he would continue to pursue FDA approval for benznidazole.

HUNTING FOR THE KISSING BUG

When I was in eighth grade, I read a library book on dream interpretation. I took notes and trained myself to read symbols, and over the years, I found I had a knack for it. I could hear a person's dream and translate the images and scenarios into information about their emotional life. The key was knowing that images are flexible. It's like reading a novel or a poem and unpacking the metaphorical meanings of broken teeth and rooms without doors.

The women in my family, however, believe in prophetic dreams. For them, dreams are screened-in porches during the summer: gathering places with loved ones. It does not matter if the person is dead. The muertos talk in dreams. Angels too. Messages are delivered in dreams, sometimes in a gesture, sometimes in whispered words, sometimes in a single image.

A year or two after Tía Dora's death, my sister phoned me. "I had a dream," Liliana said, her voice panicked. "Tía looked at me but she didn't say anything." My sister had had several dreams like this, where our auntie refused to speak to her. What could it mean?

I reached for my authoritative older sister voice and said, "You're probably needing to feel close to her." I did not share that my auntie's silence in the dream served as a painful reminder that my sister could not be in communication with her anymore.

Liliana sighed over the phone. She wanted to talk with a woman like the ones my mother and tías visited when we were growing up, a woman whose Spanish came straight from the Caribbean, whose living room boasted statues of saints and tarot cards, a woman with a booming voice and a wide neck who would hear the dream and declare, "Dora is protecting you! She is watching over you."

Such a woman would have sent us home with remedios: Place a candle next to Dora's picture. Pray the Hail Mary seven times for the soul of Dora. Crack an egg over a cup of water, and after the yolk slips into the water, write Dora's name on a piece of paper and put that in the water too.

Such rituals served as a reminder that every woman has power even against death.

...

I was not thinking about dreams when I reached College Station, Texas, and phoned Auntie Biblia in South Florida. I had told her only that I was planning to interview people about the kissing bug disease. I had not told her that I was going to spend a few hours trying to trap kissing bugs with researchers from Texas A&M University. Or that if we caught an insect, it might be infected with the parasite that had killed Tía Dora. I did not mention to my auntie that I had checked all the corners of the hotel room because kissing bugs are known to come into houses at night during the summers in Texas, as they do in Arizona and parts of the South.

"I had a dream," Auntie Biblia said. "You were eight years old and in a classroom with your book bag, and Dora was saying, 'Be careful.'"

Auntie Biblia, I understood, was anxious. I was studying the disease that had killed her sister, and dreams do not traffic in the reasonable. The common language of dreams is our fears.

But after Auntie Biblia told me her dream, I remembered my leather satchel from Colombia, which I carted around our neighborhood in New Jersey when I was in kindergarten. It had a stiff bottom and soft straps and the letters *A*, *B*, and *C* stenciled on the front in vibrant colors. I remembered the satchel and how when I was five years old I thought Tía Dora knew everything about the world.

I forgot about dream interpretation and checked that I had bought the heavy-duty bug spray. I peered under the hotel bed and in the bathroom. I recalled what the young Texas A&M research assistant had told me over the phone: the surest way to catch a kissing bug in Texas is to sit in a field when the sun falls behind the brush. The insects will come, tempted by the best possible bait—the warmth of your own body.

It was clear to me now that after visiting Professor Guhl's insect colony I had begun to change somehow. I stopped wincing when I spotted photographs of kissing bugs in science articles, and I even began looking for the images, which was how I came to know that one species of kissing bug in Central America, *Triatoma dimidiata*, often appears like an elongated copper coin with black stripes along the outer edges of its back. A species common in Texas, *Triatoma sanguisuga*, has the inverse: a dark body with reddish-orange stripes at its back's rim.

This new obsession with the bodies of kissing bugs did not strike me as odd. Grief had done stranger things to other women, pushing them into depressions and bad makeovers and beds that did not belong to them. I was merely spending the night in search of a little beast with a striped skirt.

...

The hunt for kissing bugs started at dusk on the Texas A&M College Station campus. I arrived dressed for a safari in a breathable pink button-down shirt and cargo pants with enough pockets for pens, notebooks, and my cell phone. The two research assistants, both young men in jeans and T-shirts, appeared ready for a night at the local bar. One wore cowboy boots, the other a baseball cap.

We gathered at a building that looked like a long shed. "This is bug-trapping headquarters," joked Adam Curtis, the assistant with the baseball cap. Inside, the room was narrow and well lit. Several university researchers used the room to store equipment for different studies, and the shelves were stocked with headlamps, markers, Velcro straps, and coolers. A basket on the floor teemed with light bedsheets wrapped around poles for collecting ticks. A few nets leaned against the walls for catching bats. At the back of the room, a freezer held the carcasses of dead sandhill cranes.

In a side room, what I first thought were bars of clear soap scattered across a worktable turned out to be dead kissing bugs trapped in resin: their weak legs splayed, their needle mouthparts tucked under their heads, their translucent wings gathered. The researchers planned to use these insects as educational props, to teach people how to identify kissing bugs. They were also trapping kissing bugs across the state to map where specific species are found and to see how many are actually infected with *T. cruzi*.

Adam had a narrow, solemn face and a headlamp clipped to the lip of his baseball cap. He had started trapping kissing bugs in high school when his older sister, a graduate student here, had dragged him out of Pennsylvania and brought him south for the summers. Now he was a junior and had the distinction of being one of the youngest kissing bug hunters in the United States. He preferred catching these insects by camping out. "They're like a stalker bug," he had told me earlier. "They'll come and sit on the tent 'cause they know we're there."

Adam clicked open a toolbox the color of onyx. Inside were black lights: four thin and long bulbs whose ultraviolet light would hopefully lure the bugs.

...

I had traveled to Texas A&M University at College Station because of the work of Dr. Sarah Hamer, an associate professor at the university's College of Veterinary Medicine and Biomedical Sciences. In 2013, she and her team screened more than two hundred shelter dogs across Texas and found that close to 9 percent tested positive for *T. cruzi*. In some places, like San Antonio, the number of infected dogs was closer to 14 percent. "The major takeaway, at least with canines, is that this is widespread," she told me in her office.

When—and if—the symptoms of the kissing bug disease show themselves, the dog becomes lethargic, has difficulty breathing, and develops a distended belly. It loses interest in meals and walks. A blood test can reveal antibodies to the parasite. An X-ray of the dog's chest can show the worst of it: the heart ballooning inside the body, losing its shape.

Dr. Hamer's study was not the first that had screened dogs in Texas for the kissing bug disease. In the late 1970s, the state's health department and Pan American University found a similar infection rate among stray dogs in the state's two most southern counties. Almost thirty years later, in 2008, Sonia Kjos, an entomologist at Texas A&M University, and her team published a study of dogs and the kissing bug disease in Texas that spanned more than a decade. They estimated that based on tissue samples, clinical records, and screening tests, about 20 percent of dogs in Central and South Texas had the disease. Infected dogs have also been found in Oklahoma, Louisiana, and Virginia.

Texas is large enough that you can drive more than eight hundred miles in a single direction without leaving the state. Dr. Hamer's study stood out because she found that the kissing bug disease was not limited to South Texas. The dogs in her study came from seven shelters across the state, covering almost a dozen ecoregions. Did this mean that the kissing bug disease was on the rise in Texas, or had it always been this widespread among dogs there and no one knew because researchers had not looked farther north in the state? Dr. Hamer couldn't say, but she did tell me that "we have a lot of canine Chagas. That's not happening in other states."

The disease was also being found among people who had most likely been infected from kissing bugs native to Texas. In 2015, Melissa Nolan Garcia, an epidemiologist at Baylor College of Medicine in Houston, identified five blood donors in Texas who tested positive for *T. cruzi* and who had never traveled outside of the United States. Three of the donors had EKG abnormalities usually found when the parasite has begun its attack on the heart. "It indicates that we really do have a problem," she told me during a phone interview.

I called Caryn Bern, a professor in epidemiology at the University of California, San Francisco, who has been studying the kissing bug disease for decades in both the United States and South America. She didn't think there were more cases of the disease here, only more people studying it now. "If you don't look for it, you're not going to find it," she said.

I thought about the dogs. People do not get infected with *T. cruzi* by petting an infected dog, in much the same way that we don't generally pick up the bacteria for Lyme disease from our beloved canines. However, finding a dog harboring *T. cruzi* in its body suggests that infected kissing bugs are nearby. When I started digging through medical journals, I came across a study of dogs at the veterinary medical teaching hospital at Texas A&M University at College Station. In 1987, one out of fifty-five dogs at the hospital had tested positive for *T. cruzi*. Nearly a decade later, that number had jumped to a dozen infected dogs out of seventy.

...

The Texas A&M campus spans more than five thousand acres. At dusk, I drove on empty roads, following Adam and another research assistant, Justin Bejcek. It was summer. The bulk of the students had left, and the flat land shimmered in the falling light.

We pulled up at the city's forestry center, a square one-floor building on Rock Prairie Road. Behind the building, the field sprawled before us: a stretch of open land, a mound of mulch, a long fence. I joined Adam and Justin at the back of their truck and surveyed the equipment they had packed: the black lights, the white bedsheets strapped to poles, the plastic sandwich bags, the bottle of ethanol, and the permanent markers.

Adam and Justin pinned a bedsheet to the fence and strung a second sheet between two trees, carefully hanging the black lights on the sheets. If a kissing bug flew toward the black light, it would clutch at the sheet, treating the cotton fabric as a rock, and crawl up the sheet toward the heat of the light, mistaking it for a warm body, hoping to bite whatever mammal it found there.

I followed Adam to the front of the building, where he hauled the sheet across the grass, hoping a tick would latch on for another study. He told me how one time out on a ranch he'd found the kissing bugs easily. He sat on a pile of rocks, and "two or three came out."

I checked the hem of my pants for signs of anything with six legs but found nothing except that the fabric's color looked dull from all the insect repellent I had sprayed on it earlier.

Adam tugged the sheet across the grass, and I noticed how incredibly quiet this area was. The land opened in every direction, offering itself as a canvas. How could a place this generous in its beauty be harboring the parasite that had killed Tía Dora?

...

The kissing bug disease has been in Texas for at least a thousand years. In 2003, researchers found DNA evidence of *T. cruzi* in a mummy from the Lower Pecos area near the Rio Grande River, a place known for its prehistoric rock art and earth ovens. The man had probably been in his late thirties or early forties when he died, and at the end of his life, he had a distended belly. The parasite had apparently attacked the nerve cells in his large intestine, slowing down the organ's movements, making it so that food accumulated in the man's bowels. His meals—grasshoppers and fish, mice and bats—began to gather up inside him. (Imagine soft bones piling up at the bottom of your belly.) His colon, crowded with these partially digested foods, stretched into the area between his pelvic bones and jammed against his spine. The researchers speculated that he would have been in terrible pain for weeks, maybe longer.

The man wore a strap around his waist made of deer hide and painted red. Maybe he was trying to keep his enormous belly close to him, trying to control a part of his body that had stopped making sense. He most likely died in the spring, and his people buried him with five woven mats and stone beads.

...

While Adam and Justin continued to drag the bedsheet across the fields, I swatted at mosquitoes and buttoned my shirt sleeves at the wrists. I added another layer of bug spray. The sky was beginning to turn an inky black. The sheet hanging between the trees had gathered a nocturnal community: aquatic beetles, crickets, plant hoppers, a web spinner.

We walked over to the truck, and Adam pulled out head-lamps for Justin and me. I asked, "What's considered a jackpot with trapping kissing bugs?"

"Rachel found sixty bugs in one hour," Adam said, referring to his sister.

A graduate student, Rachel Curtis-Robles had worked with Dr. Hamer to set up a program that turned ordinary Texans into "citizen scientists," instructing people on how to identify kissing bugs around their homes and catch them and ship them to the university. By 2016, they had a collection of almost two thousand bugs. Most of the participants had found the insects in dog kennels and on their patios.

An hour passed. We walked behind the building. There was a parked pickup truck and paint buckets emptied and turned over. Timed outdoor lights came on and arched across the building's garage doors. We looked and found nothing and got bored. Adam and I started watching a beetle marching up to a scorpion. I felt larger than any fear I'd ever had about insects. "We're giants in their world," I said to Adam.

"Here's one!" Justin shouted, pointing to a ledge at the back of the building. We turned off our headlamps. This kissing bug was bigger than a common beetle and flatter. It sat on the ledge like it was waiting for company. I stopped taking notes. I felt the old terror in my body, that feeling that came when I would spot a cockroach in the kitchen and yell for my mother.

"Careful," Adam told Justin. "He'll go under the ledge."

Adam retrieved a plastic sandwich bag from the truck. Justin picked up a stick, and with one quick flick of his wrist, he flung the kissing bug from the ledge to the ground and Adam scooped it up with the bag and sealed it shut. With a red marker, he wrote on the bag: "10pm, forestry center, alive, Brazos County, around building light."

It was the first time I had seen someone catch a bug and not kill it. The insect was the size of my thumb, and it cycled its black legs furiously inside the bag but managed only to flip on its back. A *Triatoma sanguisuga*, it was one of the two most common species of kissing bugs in Texas. It had orange stripes on its abdomen. I was tempted to use the word "pretty."

Justin, who was very tall, propped the empty paint bucket next to the building and peered at some insects on the wall that huddled in the shadows. No kissing bugs.

We started walking around the building, our eyes monitoring the walls for any signs of movement. Adam, a few feet ahead of us, said, "Here's one."

This kissing bug had tucked itself into a deep shadow. How had Adam seen it? It looked like a stain. He pounced on it with a sandwich bag, and as he zipped it up, Justin explained, "If you're hesitant, you can't catch it." Despite their weak legs, kissing bugs move quickly.

Justin spotted a third kissing bug, another *T. sanguisuga*, on the wall, buried in the shadows several feet above his head. The ground below us was mulch. If Justin flung it to the ground with a stick, the kissing bug would surely escape. Adam sighed. "Let's keep looking," he said. "It's not going anywhere."

I stared at Number Three. It hung on the wall, perfectly still. It was hard to believe that in such a short time, we had found three kissing bugs, any one of which might be infected with a parasite that could leave scars on a human heart.

The front of the building had brighter lights and more of the sharp pinching sounds that male crickets generate when they scrape their wings. I spotted roving beetles on the wall and a few crickets but nothing more. We checked the ledges. Then, Justin glanced upward.

A fourth kissing bug hung from the wall a few feet above the garage door. Justin, still holding a stick, nudged the insect and tossed it to the paved diveway. Adam was about to pounce when Justin said, "Let her get it."

I startled. It was a warm Texas night with the moon pinned to the black sky, and I was face-to-face with my enemy: the kissing bug. I could lean over and bag the sucker, seal it up and swing it into the back of the truck.

But I could not do it. "No, it's okay," I stammered and stepped back.

On the ground, the kissing bug stayed perfectly still with its six feeble legs, its black abdomen and orange stripes.

Adam didn't know my fears or my family history. "Hold this," he said, and just like that he handed me the plastic sandwich bags with the first two kissing bugs and scooped up Number Four. Apparently, he thought Justin's pedagogical approach—"let her get it"—was a good idea, and I was so surprised I didn't know what to say. I lifted the bags to the light, and the two kissing bugs scrambled to the corners of their respective bags, their wings tucked, their legs pedaling. I thought of desperate people knocking on doors.

The third kissing bug, the one we had left alone, still hung to the wall on a spot too high for any of us to reach. We searched for a ladder or a step stool without luck. The cricket songs grew louder. Adam and Justin looked at the insect some more. They looked at each other. They made the decision. Justin, the tallest, would serve as the bait.

Leaning against the building, he shot his left arm straight up in the air, his palm facedown on the wall. The kissing bug sat perfectly still at the edge of the light. Justin stretched his arm farther. The heat of his body would attract the insect since kissing bugs have sensors on their antennae to detect body heat.

After some time, the kissing bug shifted on the wall, clumsily, as if drunk. It headed straight for Justin's open hand.

"It's really creepy," Justin said, laughing nervously.

The kissing bug halted, apparently offended, and began walking horizontally, still a foot or so above his hand. Directly above Justin's pinky finger, it veered toward him. It had not taken offense. It had perhaps only been measuring the distance between itself and the inside of Justin's warm palm. The bug moved closer, now looking very drunk, its body less than an inch long, swaying right and left, reaching within inches of his fingers.

"You can move your hand now," Adam warned. "That's pretty close."

Justin lowered his arm. The kissing bug followed. When Justin removed his hand altogether, the kissing bug stopped, confused, a dancer in mid-step.

Adam urged, "Try to get it a little bit lower."

Justin placed his hand on the wall again and slowly dragged his palm down. The kissing bug followed. "He's missing a front leg," Justin said.

Before I could ponder kissing bugs with missing limbs, the plastic sandwich bag crinkled. Justin pulled his hand away. The kissing bug hesitated, and Justin snatched it up in the bag.

We had been out only a few hours and had already caught four kissing bugs. Later, we learned that all were infected with *T. cruzi.*

THE MILITARY'S SEARCH

The United States military began hunting for kissing bugs in 1964 when a graduate student from Oklahoma State University, Warren Floyd Pippin, started his two-year study of the bugs at the Lackland Air Force Base in San Antonio. The work was not easy. Pippin hauled shovels, machetes, and trowels. He cleared away a cactus and dug up wood rat nests. He plucked kissing bugs from the nests and dropped them into empty ice cream cartons. Then he walked the insects back to his lab at the military base.

There, Pippin created fake wood rat nests in an outdoor cage and studied close to seven hundred kissing bugs belonging to three species. Two species, *T. gerstaeckeri* and *T. sanguisuga*, were common in Texas and the species *R. prolixus* was from South America. Pippin observed how the insects fed and how they reproduced and how quickly they molted. He noted whether they had a preference for the blood of armadillos or baby white mice or squirrels. He tracked the number of eggs the females laid over their lifetimes: anywhere between 151 and more than a thousand, depending on the species, temperature and humidity. He checked the fecal matter of each kissing bug to learn if the insect was harboring *T. cruzi*. By his count, about 78 percent of his kissing bugs were infected with the parasite.

Researchers today do not have to spend their days inspecting an insect's fecal droppings for evidence of *T. cruzi*. They have the technology to check the kissing bug's DNA. In 2012, the US military published a study showing that of the 140 kissing bugs collected on military bases in the San Antonio area, only 16 percent were found to be infected. This number struck me as very low. When Dr. Hamer and her team tested almost two thousand kissing bugs collected by Texans, more than 60 percent were infected with *T. cruzi*.

I was still wondering if Texas was seeing a rise in the number of infected kissing bugs or only a rise in the number of experts like Dr. Hamer who were searching for them. I realized it was time to call the military and find out what they knew.

...

San Antonio has a public library with a collection dedicated to works of Latinx authors. It has a culinary school and an old brewery that's been converted into a pricey hotel. In 2018, it also had the highest rate of poverty among large metro areas in the country, and as of 2013, close to 14 percent of the dogs in the city's shelters were infected with *Trypanosoma cruzi*.

It is also in the San Antonio area at the Lackland Air Force Base where the Defense Department trains its military dogs—the ones that patrol airports, sniff out explosives in Iraq, and prowl through Afghanistan, like the dog that was airlifted into Osama bin Laden's compound in Pakistan in 2011. The base also houses the Defense Department's veterinary hospital for military dogs.

If a dog is wounded on a mission, it returns to San Antonio for surgeries, for veterinary care, for rehab.

The military dogs typically train for four months at Lackland and then work for at least a decade before they are retired. A great deal of federal money is involved. "A fully trained military dog costs about as much as a small missile," a Bloomberg journalist reported. In 2016, the military had approximately 1,800 dogs in service. A retired dog handler told the *San Antonio Express-News* that with training and care, every military dog is worth between $80,000 and $100,000.

Uno was one of those dogs. When the director of the military's veterinary services, Colonel Cheryl Sofaly, began telling me about him over the phone, I immediately pictured a German shepherd, a long snout and soft ears, a personality bold enough to be named number one.

Colonel Sofaly said Uno's training was going well. He was two years old and healthy. Then one day, Uno's handler opened the dog's kennel, but Uno bounced out and collapsed. The trainer picked him up and ran him straight to the ICU. "He was in cardiac arrest," the colonel explained. An ultrasound of Uno's chest showed the familiar signs of the kissing bug disease: his canine heart enlarged. The organ was riddled with *T. cruzi.*

No one knew how Uno had gotten the parasite. Maybe he spotted a kissing bug that had crawled into his kennel and ate it or just as likely a kissing bug fed on Uno during the night. It was not the first time a military dog had suffered from the kissing bug disease.

In the late seventies, a Labrador retriever at Lackland developed a strange, distended belly. The veterinarians put him down, and when they sliced open the Lab's chest, they found that part of the dog's heart had lost its shape. The right ventricle was "flabby and dilated," according to a published report. The veterinarians found the parasite lodged in the dog's cardiac tissue.

The finding did not spur the military to start testing its dogs for the kissing bug disease, but in 2006, that all changed. Veterinarians at Lackland began reporting more cases of what's called canine Chagas disease. Testing revealed that 8 percent of the military dogs at one base were infected, which is similar to what Dr. Hamer found among shelter dogs across the state.

Over the next decade, the military identified the parasite in seventy of their dogs, Colonel Sofaly told me. And so she and her colleagues began battling the kissing bug—cutting back shrubs around kennels, installing screens, and spraying pesticides farther into the brush.

Are the dogs retired when they're diagnosed? "If they're not symptomatic, they can do any duty," Colonel Sofaly said, except for work with the Transportation Security Administration, which brings dogs into contact with the public. Even though these dogs would not themselves generally pose a risk to people, it would be a public relations problem.

What about the people who train at Lackland?

About thirty-five thousand recruits come through the air force base, Dr. Thomas Cropper told me when we spoke in 2016. A veterinarian, he was the primary epidemiologist for trainees at the base, and he was worried because recruits were sent out on the base for a week or two at a time. The Texas landscape with its heat and sand and brush simulates the geography of the Middle East. Dr. Cropper and his team had taken new measures against the kissing bugs: spraying the recruits' tents with insecticides, stressing the use of insect repellents among trainees, and giving them bed netting. "You don't want to cause panic, but you don't want to ignore something you could do a lot about," he said.

Between 2014 and 2016, the military screened more than forty thousand service members at the base for the kissing bug disease and confirmed that only two people tested positive. Both service members had grown up in Texas. They included an eighteen-year-old who already had early heart disease—a cardiac MRI showed the parasite had attacked his left ventricle. He'd spent his childhood on a ranch, where he had seen the kissing bugs in his family's home. In another nine recruits, the tests were inconclusive.

Apparently, even if the number of infected kissing bugs was growing in Texas, the insects were not posing a significant risk to people.

...

At Cropper's suggestion, I phoned Dr. Roy Madigan, a veterinarian near San Antonio, who told me that he saw more kissing bugs now than when he first moved to the area close to twenty years ago. It didn't matter that his house was in the suburbs or that it had the kind of modern windows meant to block all insects. The kissing bugs still managed to crawl inside. "My wife found one in her purse on her iPhone," he said, laughing at the absurdity.

I remembered reading about a family in Central Texas who reported the same observation to the CDC. After living in the exact same location for thirteen years, the family had started to see kissing bugs for the first time around 2007. They had fifteen dogs on their ranch, and one died from the kissing bug disease. Seven other dogs were infected. The family noticed this uptick around the same time that the military began screening for the disease in their dogs at Lackland Air Force Base.

Dr. Madigan believed the disease was on the rise in Texas for a simple reason: "we are developing more land." Starting in the late nineties, Texas had more than a million acres of open land turned over for development, and between 2010 and 2017, it had added more housing than any other state—close to a million units. In 2018, Apple announced it was building a $1 billion campus in the Austin area on a former ranch that measures about seven thousand acres.

Dr. Madigan looked at the state's housing boom from the kissing bug's perspective. In Texas, these insects feed on mammals like wood rats. The housing boom was disrupting that ecological process, and more housing translates into more families with pet dogs. To the kissing bug, those dogs are no different from wood rats, Dr. Madigan said. The dogs are dinner. "It's like having baby wood rats in your backyard," he told me.

And what about climate change? Was it affecting kissing bugs?

Insects that carry disease are usually sensitive to temperature shifts. Warmer temperatures can change how often a mosquito bites a person, and kissing bugs tend to feed more frequently during warmer times of the year. That said, scientists have pointed out that it is hard to isolate climate change as the single cause for the spread of vector-borne diseases. There are too many other factors to consider including housing conditions, access to healthcare, and land development. Also while insects carrying pathogens might appear in a new area when it becomes warmer, they could die off in another area that grows too hot.

A few studies on the possible effects of climate change on the kissing bug disease have turned up varying results. In Chile, one group of researchers mapped the risk of the parasite being transmitted from one common triatomine species called *T. infestans* and found that climate change could increase the risk of transmission in certain parts of the country. Argentinian researchers looked at five species of kissing bugs in Venezuela and found that higher temperatures would make certain regions of that country less friendly to the insects, though their model did not consider the risk for transmission of the parasite.

In 2013, researchers from the University of Texas-Pan American and the University of Texas at Austin teamed up with colleagues from Mexico's Universidad Nacional Autónoma and focused on predicting how climate change might alter the fate of two species of the kissing bugs common in Texas: *T. sanguisuga* and *T. gerstaeckeri*. One model showed the insects moving as far north as Michigan and New York.

...

In 2015, the CDC granted Texas researchers a half-million-dollar federal grant, spread out over five years, to raise awareness among health care providers about the kissing bug disease. It was part of an initiative to tackle a handful of what the CDC labeled "neglected parasitic infections." Dr. Susan Montgomery, who leads the epidemiology team at the CDC's parasitic diseases branch and is a leading expert on the kissing bug disease in the United States, told me, "We consider them neglected because there's relatively little attention that's been devoted to their surveillance or prevention or treatment in the US."

The list of neglected parasitic infections includes the kissing bug disease and also toxoplasmosis—the disease that made news when Martin Shkreli hiked the price on a drug used to treat it. Also on the list: toxocariasis, a disease caused by dog and cat roundworms, and most common among poor Black people in the US. Every year, the disease blinds at least seventy people, most of them children.

How did a half-million-dollar federal grant for the kissing bug disease end up in Texas? Dr. Cropper from the Lackland Air Force Base told me it was, in part, because he brought the opportunity to the attention of Paula Stigler Granados, a professor in public health, who at the time was teaching at the University of Texas's regional campus in San Antonio. Professor Stigler Granados applied for the five-year grant, received it, and created the Texas Chagas Task Force, connecting veterinarians, health professionals, and entomologists across the state. Its members produced a guide to kissing bugs in Texas and a video for health care providers, and when the CDC funding fell short after a few years, Professor Stigler Granados applied for local grants and got them.

Another CDC grant was awarded to Morven Edwards, a pediatric infectious disease specialist in Texas, who created educational materials about the congenital form of the kissing bug disease and who gave grand rounds, or medical lectures, about it.

There was only one problem with the federal government sending money for the kissing bug disease to Texas: it is not where most infected people live. A year after the grants were announced, a study led by Jennifer Manne-Goehler, a clinical fellow at Harvard Medical School, estimated that California has about seventy thousand people with the kissing bug disease—all of whom, like Tía Dora, are immigrants from Latin America. This number of people surpasses that in every other state in the country, including Texas, which has only about half the number of infections.

Dr. Montgomery at the CDC couldn't answer my questions about funding. She did explain that there had been an application process and a review of those applications, and I realized that the agency had not proactively directed the money toward Texas as much as it had reacted to applications from the state. Dr. Montgomery also insisted that these measures had made a difference across the country in raising awareness of the disease.

"When blood screening started in 2007 in the United States, we would get calls from health care providers whose patients showed up in their office with a letter from the blood bank saying: 'You tested positive for Chagas disease,'" Dr. Montgomery said. "Now, this year, most of the inquiries are from providers whose patient is an immigrant from Latin America."

...

No one I spoke to thought Americans had to worry about an outbreak of the kissing bug disease from insects native to the United States. The CDC has recorded fewer than a hundred such infections. Even if these bugs managed to colonize a suburban home, pesticides are usually easy to find at local stores and often affordable. Also, a worried person can contact local health officials, perhaps sooner than one seventy-four-year-old woman did in rural Louisiana a year after Hurricane Katrina. She had more than fifty bites from kissing bugs, and streaks of fecal matter from the insects could be seen on the walls of her house. After a fumigation, twenty dead kissing bugs were collected. While more than half the insects carried *T. cruzi*, and the woman herself tested positive, this remains a rare case.

A more common scenario is what occurred in Arizona between 2017 and 2018. Researchers screened more than a hundred women and men in Tuscon and Bisbee who reported bites from local kissing bugs, and while they found that some people had allergic reactions to the bites, not a single person turned up infected with *T. cruzi*.

IF TÍA HAD KNOWN

If I had told my auntie that I planned to gaze, in person, upon the parasite *T. cruzi*, she would have startled and asked, "Is it really possible to look at it?" She would have grimaced, pulled her shoulders up to her ears, as if the news offended her. She would have turned into a journalist: Where will you see it? With whom? Is it safe? Are you sure it's safe?

Tía Dora would have asked all this from the sofa in her living room, her feet tucked under her as if she were a schoolgirl and not a woman in her late fifties. Though I knew it was the disease that made her look tiny and delicate, I sometimes blamed the furniture in her apartment. The entertainment center spanned a wall of the living room and a television set crowded another wall, and after Tío Papeles died, Tía Dora placed a dining table into that same room. Sometimes weighing only eighty pounds, my auntie looked like she lived in a dollhouse stuffed with too much furniture.

She was not a timid woman though. It was one trait that we shared. We were both driven. She had wanted to become a schoolteacher in the United States and had barreled her way through bureaucracy and college courses in English do that. And me? I wanted to know what had killed her and what had terrified me, and so one afternoon, I called a complete stranger who had spent a lifetime studying the parasite *T. cruzi* and asked if he would answer a few questions and if I could see the parasites he had worked with. He said yes. I only had to make my way to Iowa.

...

Dr. Louis Kirchhoff was waiting for me at the airport in Cedar Rapids. He immediately reminded me of the older editors at the *New York Times*, where I reported for a year during my twenties. He had a carefully trimmed white beard and carried a small notebook and several pens in his shirt pocket. He looked like a reporter ready to find a good story.

I had tracked his work for more than a year. Often, Dr. Kirchhoff's name popped up in articles about testing people for the kissing bug disease. In the mid-eighties, having finished medical school and a four-year fellowship at the National Institutes of Health, he took a position as an assistant professor at the University of Iowa and began, as he told me, "pushing around strands of DNA" from *T. cruzi*.

Three decades later, discussing the prospect of this trip, he had told me, "It'll be fun. You'll like the parasite."

...

Confession: initially, I found it easier to look at photographs of *Trypanosoma cruzi* than the kissing bugs. The insects felt familiar and horrifying while the single-celled parasite—magnified and photographed—struck me as something I would find in an

Octavia Butler science fiction novel, which is to say that *T. cruzi* is a shape-shifter. In the belly of a kissing bug, it looks like a tadpole with a pointed face and is called an epimastigote. When the parasite moves into the insect's lower intestines, it takes on the appearance of an eel with a Mohawk—a trypomastigote. In that form, the parasite leaves the kissing bug by way of the insect's feces, and when it has the fortune to land upon a human body, particularly near a person's eyes, mouth, or nose, it invades.

Its shape-shifting is not done. Once *T. cruzi* makes it into the human body, it penetrates cells, and after a few hours, it turns into what can be described as a lavender coin: an oval shape, the tail almost gone, and, often in stained slides, with a lavender hue. In this stage, the parasite is now an amastigote and begins to multiply. This can happen in the tissue of the human heart. The lavender coin becomes two, then four, and so on, and after several cycles, the parasites shape-shift again, this time back into eels with Mohawks. They vibrate. They thrash. They overwhelm the cell they inhabit, killing it in the process, and the parasites begin hunting again—finding another cell, sneaking in, and transforming again into coins. If this cycle is repeated often enough in the heart, cells gradually die off, and scar tissue forms. Over the course of decades, the heart loses strength. It is hard to pump blood with scar tissue.

The parasite is technically a trypanosome. From the Greek, *trypanon* means a borer, one that punctures wood or plant material by rotating. *Soma* means body. An organism that drills into the body. The term *trypanosome* was actually coined in 1843 when a scientist first found the parasite in frogs.

...

During lunch near Iowa City, Dr. Kirchhoff explained, over his margarita pizza, that *T. cruzi* has a special pouch of DNA minicircles called a kinetoplast. "It's loaded with DNA," he said, adding that the RNA messages transcribed from the DNA undergo a lot of editing, which raises many questions. "Why do they have a complicated system for editing messages? We don't do that, and we're more complicated."

He told me that once the parasite makes its way into the human body, it has a lot to consider. "Here's the problem. From the parasite's perspective, as soon as they get in, they get attacked by the immune system." Millions of years ago, though, the parasite figured out a way around this issue: it exits the bloodstream. "What *T. cruzi* does is get into the cells and multiply, and they don't have to deal with attacks."

In other words, the parasite finds a sanctuary in the human body, where it can reproduce safely. I thought this was cunning, but Dr. Kirchhoff did not approve of that word, arguing that it has a negative connotation. "They're very smart," he said between bites of pizza, and technically *T. cruzi* is not targeting humans. It takes up residence in a great number of mammal species. Again, from the parasite's perspective, humans just happen to be another mammal.

Dr. Kirchhoff spent years trying to figure out how to test people for evidence of *T. cruzi* infection. Along with his collaborator Keiko Otsu, he recombined distinct segments of the parasite's DNA to create hybrid coding sequences. They inserted these hybrids into benign laboratory strains of *E. coli*. These bacteria functioned like factories, churning out billions of the hybrid re-combinant proteins derived from *T. cruzi*. After much testing, Dr. Kirchhoff and Otsu figured out which of these hybrid recom-binant proteins would work best in testing people for the kissing bug disease.

He licensed the proteins to Abbott Diagnostics, and by 2016, the FDA had approved three tests for screening blood donors across the country, including two that primarily use Dr. Kirchhoff's hybrid recombinant proteins. If a blood donor is in-fected with *T. cruzi*, some of the donor's antibodies will recognize these recombinant proteins and grab on to them. "These bound antibodies can then be detected," Dr. Kirchhoff noted, and this leads to a positive test result.

...

The day clouded over as Dr. Kirchhoff and I walked across the University of Iowa campus toward the Eckstein Medical Research Building. It was here that he had worked for so many years with *T. cruzi*'s DNA. While Dr. Kirchhoff was no longer conducting new research, he kept batches of the parasite on hand to meet federal regulations for the screening test and borrowed lab space from a generous colleague in the building.

The laboratory had steel-gray counters, rows of sterilized flasks, and lots of binders stuffed with papers. Dr. Kirchhoff hauled what looked like a Styrofoam cooler from off the top of a metal shelf and carried it into a room with two biosafety cabinets and a table with two microscopes. He pulled a flask from the cooler and held it to the light. It looked like it had a shot of bourbon in it. The liquid was a suspension of bovine liver powder and salts, and I could see dots floating in it: *T. cruzi*—millions, alive.

Dr. Kirchhoff rocked the flask so the liquid spread. "They think they're in the gut of an insect," he said. In other words, the parasites didn't know they were in a flask. They thought they were inside a kissing bug.

These parasites, Dr. Kirchhoff told me, belonged to the Tulahuén strain, which has been widely studied by scientists conducting research into *T. cruzi*. It was isolated from a person who lived in Tulahuén, Chile, during the 1940s, and it had been maintained in liquid culture all these decades. In other words, I was in a room with the descendants of parasites that had been isolated from someone in South America before Tía Dora was born.

I noticed a flask in the cooler labeled "LOL." "What does that stand for?"

"Lots of life," he said, matter-of-fact.

He put the flask under the microscope, adjusted the lenses, and after a few seconds, he declared, "This is the best. It's just loaded with parasites."

I laughed to avoid feeling the fear in my gut, and I peered into the microscope. At first, I saw a blurry piece of white paper. When my eyes adjusted, I noticed clumps of tangled black hair floating into view. Besides the thin, tangled hair strands, pencil marks stained the screen, as if a child had drawn the number one sideways, vertically, and diagonally. The more I looked at the field visible through the microscope, the more the flask of parasites reminded me of a cell phone, its screen cracked and scratched. Where were the parasites? "I can't see it," I finally said.

Dr. Kirchhoff adjusted the microscope. When I still couldn't make out the parasite, he patiently pulled out his iPhone, took a photo of the flask, then zoomed in. "There," he said, satisfied. "You can see them now."

I squinted at the photograph. "Wait. The scratches are the parasites?" I asked, dumbfounded.

Dr. Kirchhoff examined the photograph on his phone. He had studied this parasite for much of his professional life. They were apparently as familiar to him as his own fingernails, and I had just told him the object of his obsession looked like a scratched cell phone screen. "I guess you could say that," he said hesitantly.

I returned to the microscope. I focused my eyes on one area of the flask, and this time I could see that the scratch on the glass was thrashing. Its tail, or flagellum, enabled the parasite to move. I focused on a second scratch, another parasite. This one floated, the movement so incredibly slight, it would be easy to miss. I watched as a third parasite joined a tangle of fine black hair. My vision shifted, and I could see that the clump of fine hair was not a clump at all, but rather a bundle of parasites, their tails vibrating.

...

Another confession: I did not think of Tía Dora when I saw the parasites. I watched them thrash and thought: They're alive. They are tinier than a strand of human hair, and they are alive. Later, I wondered how I could have been taken, even for a few seconds, by a shape-shifting parasite that can kill the human heart and that had killed my auntie.

IN SEARCH OF
OTHER FAMILIES

FALTA

Tía Dora would have approved of my new life in Ohio, and specifically my apartment. She would have liked the hardwood floors, the built-in bookshelves, and the elm tree outside the living room window. She would have loved the park around the corner, the coffee and quiche sold on the main street, and the shopkeeper who imported gloves knitted in Peru. She would have admired the historic gas lamps on the sidewalk, then told my mother on the phone that the apartment was "del high class."

She would have adored the college campus where I was teaching, swelled with pride when I told her the school had opened in the early nineteenth century, taken pictures with me next to the red-brick buildings. She would have raised both eyebrows when I told her that civil rights activists trained college students here in 1964 to register Black voters in Mississippi. She would have murmured, "Tiene su historia," which would have been her polite Colombian way of acknowledging that key historical events had taken place, but she never wanted to be involved in anything political.

She would have adored the Queen Anne dining table I bought, the stylish curve of the table's legs, the gleaming cherry-wood, the newly upholstered seats. She would have sat there with me in the evening during a long weekend visit and debated aloud if she dared to eat more of the pasta I had cooked for us.

...

I am lying to myself.

Tía Dora would never have visited me in Ohio. She would have stopped talking to me shortly after I moved here when it became clear that I had a new sweetheart and that my sweetheart was not a cisgender man. Tía would have realized that "amistad" was the word I used for several months to avoid gendering my sweetheart in Spanish, and she would have grown suspicious when I referred to my sweetheart as "amiga" while my sister called my sweetie "amigo."

Maybe she would have come to my sister's wedding in a silk dress and heels, sat at a different table, and ignored my sweetheart and me. She would have poked at the rice during the reception, danced some but not to the Ricky Martin songs, which she thought were ridiculous. Or maybe she would have refused to attend the wedding, but I doubt it. I want to doubt it. I want to think Tía Dora loved my sister so much it would have made everything else, including who I loved, tolerable for an afternoon.

...

In Spanish, absence is ausencia, and also the word falta, whose definition spreads across two pages of the Spanish-English dictionary that once belonged to Tía Dora and is now mine. Falta is a noun, a verb, an adjective. It means the absence of pesos, the not having enough milk, the needing más de todo. It means a transgression in soccer, the penalty for kicking or tripping or shoving another player. It can mean a love that is not here, as in: "me haces falta," or "I miss you" which I always hear as: "you make me miss you."

...

The more I interviewed experts on the kissing bug disease, the more I returned to a memory of Tía Dora. It was the summer of 2000, just before I'd come out to my family as bisexual; the summer that Tía Dora spent two straight months in the hospital with her esophagus dilated again.

When I arrived at the hospital in the middle of that summer, I found the curtain partly drawn around her bed. Tía Dora was so thin, so fragile, that she looked like a bird with broken wings. She must have weighed less than ninety pounds.

She tried to smile. I leaned over to kiss her forehead. She raised her right hand to touch my shoulder.

"Me hicistes falta," she whispered and began crying.

My throat tightened. We were not a family that said, "I love you," that cried openly, that said, "I miss you," which was what Tía was telling me. She had missed me. It was the closest she ever came to saying, "I love you."

In that moment, she was not the auntie who had banished me from her life when I came out to my family; she was not the auntie who had cared more about appearances than about me. She was the tía who said, "Me hicistes falta."

I held this memory of Tía Dora like an amulet, a protection against the part of her that had hated me. Also, without this memory, my grief did not make sense to me.

...

I spent most of that summer in 2000 next to Tía Dora's hospital bed. We watched television. I flipped through magazines and showed her pictures of celebrities. When we ran out of gossip about family members, we moved on to friends, then las vecinas. I napped or she did. Auntie Biblia and my mother took turns on the other side of the bed. We never left her alone. At night, Auntie Biblia slept in the chair or in the other hospital bed when it was empty.

One afternoon, Tía Dora told Auntie Biblia not to be silly. "Vayas y descanses," Tía Dora said, and she pointed out that I was there with her and Auntie Biblia should go home and take a good shower and rest, stop at the church if she wanted.

Auntie Biblia hesitated. She was fifty-nine that year, and I was twenty-five, and she looked me in the face for a long time, thinking about whether or not she could trust me with Tía Dora.

I said, "Go, Tía. I'm here. Nada va a pasar."

Finally she left, and a short time later, Tía Dora needed to use the bathroom. We rang for an orderly and waited. No one came. "I can take you," I said and started to help Tía out of the bed.

She had lost so much weight that it felt like I was assisting a young child. I placed my hand under her right forearm, and she quickly grabbed it, unsteady on her feet. Upright, she dragged her slippers on the floor softly, and after a few steps she stopped, glanced at me, and started giggling. Using my childhood nickname of Tata, she said, "Tata is taking me to the bathroom." She giggled again. I said, "That's right," as if I had been this grown up for a long time. Slowly, we made our way.

JANET AND HER BABY

Tía Dora tried to have children. When I learned this after she died, it surprised me. She had us. That was my first thought, as if my sister and I should have been all the children she and Tío Papeles wanted or needed. I had chosen not to have any, and I had figured that Tía had done the same. She had not. She had wanted a baby, her own child, but pregnancy had eluded her.

Her body, of course, would have struggled with a pregnancy, and I don't think she knew that the parasite for the kissing bug disease can jump from mother to baby in utero. It's called congenital Chagas disease, and it can be hard to identify because infected newborns can be born prematurely and have symptoms like jaundice and anemia, which are easily attributed to other causes.

Such a transmission happened in Washington, DC, around 1985. Dr. Kirchhoff, who was working at the National Institutes of Health at the time, screened more than two hundred people—all of whom had grown up in Central America—for the kissing bug disease. Almost 5 percent of the people screened in the study had the disease. One, however, had been born in the United

143

States: a three-month-old baby whose mother, like mine, was an immigrant. The baby was infected.

The CDC estimates that anywhere between 63 and 315 babies infected with *T. cruzi* are born every year in the United States. In Latin America, the numbers are much higher: an estimated nine thousand children are infected in utero each year.

I thought of these children in the United States as "lost babies." The CDC and state public health officials do not know who they are because pregnant women are not routinely screened for the kissing bug disease in this country. If they were, many of the lost babies could be saved since the drug benznidazole can often cure children with the disease. But lost babies cannot be treated. According to the Pan American Health Organization, about one-third of all new infections with *T. cruzi* come from mother-to-child transmission.

Sometimes these lost babies are not found until they are grown. In 2013, a man in his early twenties showed up in an emergency room in Miami with chest pains. His lab results and EKG were normal. A year later, he tested positive for the kissing bug disease when he donated blood. His brother, two years older, also tested positive. Born and raised in the United States, they were infected in utero. The parasite had spared the older brother's heart but attacked the younger brother's, interfering with its electrical currents, making it so that he had irregular heartbeats.

...

I scoured medical literature and found one baby who had not been lost. In 2010, the year Tía Dora died, a boy in Virginia was born prematurely at twenty-nine weeks. He weighed just a little more than four pounds and fluids were building up in his chest cavity that could damage his heart and lungs. When his mother told doctors that she had the kissing bug disease but had never received treatment, they tested samples of the baby's blood and found the trypomastigote form of *T. cruzi.* The parasite was circulating in his body, looking for cells to invade. Treated with benznidazole, the baby was free of the parasite within a year. When I phoned the pediatrician, though, she told me the family didn't want to talk to the media. Unfortunately, I was the media.

I continued interviewing experts about the kissing bug disease, and one day, a cardiologist told me about a mother named Janet who had the disease and was willing to speak with me. Janet agreed to talk with me because she hoped that if I wrote her story, the pesadilla, the nightmare, would not happen to another family.

I agreed to protect her privacy, not to publish pictures of her and her family, and after the 2016 presidential election, I decided not to use her last name and to avoid, as much as possible, references to her country of origin because I could not be sure, now, what anyone would do with that information.

...

When I met Janet, I was immediately taken with her house in Maryland. She and her husband had landscaped the front yard and started installing a white picket fence. The front door was a deep shade of cranberry. The pavement on the driveway gleamed. I took one look at her house and thought: this is a woman who wants a good life. I thought, too, of Tía Dora, the striver immigrant, the luchadora immigrant. Somehow this was all there in the cranberry door and the start of that picket fence.

Janet, in her late thirties, looked like the actress Sofía Vergara without the spiky heels. She had long wavy hair and almond-shaped eyes. The day we met, she pulled her hair into a bun, and she spoke to me intimately, as if we had known each other all our lives. She addressed her family members with love: "mi amor," "mi niño." She was delighted that I had noticed the details of her home. "You should have seen how it looked!" she said, smiling proudly as she told me about the changes they'd made to the house. They had cleared not only shrubs from their yard but seven giant trees and what felt to her like miles of poison ivy. She had insisted on clearing the yard so she could one day look out the front window and see her children playing in the sun.

We sat on the brown sofa in her living room, and she told me how the nightmare began.

. . .

It had been the spring of 2015, and the day started with lipstick and mascara. Janet felt good. Fabulous, really. Mother's Day had recently passed and she was pregnant with her second son. Her due date was not until August. She had plenty of time. She applied her makeup that morning and tucked her long hair, the color of caramel, under a turquoise summer hat. She dressed her two-year-old son, Junior, in a crisp pair of shorts and shiny sneakers. Her husband, José, worked long hours on construction sites, and she loved that he had the day off. Their friends, another couple with a toddler, joined them. They were all driving to New York City for the day and stopping for lunch in Ocean City, about three hours from their home.

On the boardwalk, the vendors' voices spiraled in the air, and Janet and her husband and their friends took pictures and ordered lunch. It was American food: pasta dishes and beef. They told jokes and laughed and kept their eyes on the children. Then, with no warning, Janet felt a seeping between her legs. Was it urine? Her underwear grew wet. She panicked. "I need the bathroom," she told her husband and friends, and she sprang from the table and hurried through the crowd on the boardwalk, trying to get to a public restroom. Her underwear now felt completely soaked. Her black stretch pants too. Her breathing quickened.

She pushed faster across the boardwalk, past the families squealing on four-seated bicycles. José kept in quick step next to her with their friends and the children. Janet had already been to the hospital earlier that week. Her body had not felt right. Some days the baby hardly moved. Almost every day, she felt her belly slightly harden, the muscles stiffen, an orange that refused to be squeezed. At the hospital, they had taken her blood pressure and checked the baby's heartbeat. A nurse had explained that everything was normal. That if she didn't feel the baby move at all, she should come back. That if anything changed, she should come back. Now her underwear was drenched and her black stretch pants too. What was happening?

Janet pushed the bathroom door open and went in with her friend María while the men waited outside with the children. In the bathroom, Janet shut the stall door behind her. She pulled down her pants. She couldn't make out a color on the dark fabric. She wiped, then cried out to María, "It's blood!"

She wiped again. The blood soiled the toilet paper, red and bright.

María, on the other side of the stall door, murmured, "Tranquila, tranquila."

Janet wiped again and the blood did not stop.

From the other side of the stall's door, María tempered her voice and said, "Janet, roll up the toilet paper. Make a pad."

Janet yanked on the toilet roll, piling the sheets in her hands.

Outside, she said to José, "We need to find a hospital. I'm bleeding."

...

The next ten hours crushed together in confusion.

They arrived at one hospital near the beach, but the doctors sent her to another hospital. Janet didn't understand. All the words ran together in English. She didn't speak the language, but José did. From what he could understand, the other hospital had a better-equipped maternity ward.

The bleeding slowed. The bleeding stopped. At the second hospital, a doctor said Janet would need to stay for observation. José told her, "We're three hours from home. What if you have the baby here? We don't have anyone here."

The thought of a birth felt impossible. It was May, not August. The calendar couldn't collapse, not like this. But what if José was right? What if the baby came? Tomorrow or in a few days? At least in Maryland they had his auntie and a circle of friends. Everyone else—their parents, Janet's sisters—lived in South America.

Janet was worried, too, about Junior. Her two-year-old had wailed from his father's arms when the ambulance had taken her to the second hospital. He needed a proper meal, a bath. Under the fluorescent hospital lights, Janet dressed.

It was after ten at night. They drove south on 95, the highway unfurling in the night, pointing toward home. The next morning, they drove to the hospital where Janet received her prenatal care. The baby looked fine on the monitors. Everything was normal. The doctors sent her home, insisting on total bed rest.

But Janet had been pregnant before. This did not feel the same. The hardness of her belly, the way that hardness came and went, bothered her. She looked for comfort in what the women back home had told her: all pregnancies are different. She hoped they were right.

...

Hearing Janet's story, I tried to remember that the numbers are low. At most, 315 babies are born infected with *T. cruzi* every year in the United States, and only a few of those babies will grow up to have heart damage. A smaller percentage of those babies with heart problems will die. And yet the longer that I held Janet's story, the more difficult it became to think of numbers—one lost baby is impossible to bear.

...

A few days after their Ocean City trip, José woke up at four in the morning to drive to the construction site. He kissed Janet goodbye in the dark, and she ambled through the house, grateful that Junior was still sleeping. She made her way to the sofa, beneath framed family portraits. Already Junior had grown so much. In one photograph, he was not yet a year old, dressed in a sailor's outfit, a chubby-faced boy with his father's eyes. Janet rested on the sofa, her hair a long coil around her shoulders.

Janet had not planned on having children in the United States—in fact, she had not expected to live in this country. The youngest of nine children, she had grown up in South America where she had seen her mother make do with very little and had watched an older sister stay in an abusive marriage. One day, Janet looked at her mother and sister and vowed that she would never be taken advantage of by any man, neither with a slap to the face nor by legal means in court. With the help of her older siblings, she graduated from law school. She landed a legal job in the city and started making money. Good money. While her coworkers vacationed in the United States, Janet took her mother on day trips in their own country, indulging the old woman with gifts: earrings, new lipstick, a generous lunch.

Periodically friends asked who she was dating, but Janet waved them away. "I don't have time," she'd say. In her thirties, she lived with her mom and used her savings to buy houses, fix them up, and rent them out. Once a girl from a family of modest means, Janet planned on becoming a landowner.

Then one day, a friend declared, "I've met your soul mate, Janet. He's just like you. He only works and thinks of his mom. If I wasn't already with someone, I'd have him for myself."

José lived in the suburbs of Washington, DC. He drove cranes on construction sites and called his mother in South

America with a duty verging on obsession. Money was the reason he had come to the United States at eighteen, and more than a decade later, José worked twelve- to fourteen-hour days and had savings and two cars. He had picked up plenty of English, too, enough to hold conversations and pass his citizenship test, and for a time, he had run his own carpet-cleaning company. When a friend of his sister's pushed Janet's phone number into his hand, he called. That first time, they stayed on the phone for hours.

No one was more surprised than Janet. They began speaking on the phone every day. One afternoon, José called and said, "Open your front door." He had sent his sister with a CD of romantic ballads. Another time, he arranged for the delivery of a cake and flowers. Soon, the bachelor who had expected to grow old alone in Maryland was talking of marriage, and three months after meeting over the phone, they did marry. Janet wore a strapless dress and gloves the color of new pearls. She moved to Maryland. She became pregnant with Junior. She looked around at their basement apartment one day and declared, "We need a house, José. We can't raise a family in a basement."

They found the house in Maryland covered with trees and shrubs. It was in a county that had once been home only to white and Black families. By 2014, when Janet and her husband moved into the house, about a quarter of the public school students in the county came from Latinx families.

Now Janet had doctor's orders to rest until the baby arrived, but she didn't know how she was supposed to be on bed rest and taking care of a toddler at the same time. She spent the morning moving between Junior and the sofa. She gave him a bottle of milk and went back to the sofa. She changed his diaper and returned to the sofa. Then, the contractions started. The pain ripped across her back and her belly.

José called every half hour to check in. "I'm having pain," she said.

"Do you want me to come home?"

"No, I'm okay."

By eleven, the contractions came with furious intensity. She phoned José and said, "I have to go to the hospital."

...

In the emergency room, the overhead lights jumped at Janet, and so did the English questions. José stayed in the waiting room with Junior because toddlers were not allowed into the exam room. Janet kept her cell phone on so he could hear everything the staff was saying and interpret. After the nurse left and Janet hung up the phone, she closed her eyes. A wetness ran between her legs, the liquid warm against her thighs. It turned into a river. Where was everyone?

A nurse appeared. Janet whispered, "Everything's wet." She could feel the gurney's mattress soaked beneath her, but felt too weak to move. The nurse lifted the hospital sheet, then immediately dropped it and ran from the room. Janet was hemorrhaging. Nurses and doctors arrived frantic. All Janet could think of was her baby, that the doctors needed to save her baby, that her body mattered only to the degree that it held her baby. Her body was a purse she could mend later.

The baby had begun to leave her, the placenta peeling away.

In the operating room, a nurse cradled Janet's head and murmured, "You're okay, Mami. You're okay."

Janet didn't answer. She closed her eyes. She couldn't be having the baby. It was too early.

The nurse rubbed her cheek. "Stay awake, Mami. Stay awake."

. . .

Luis was born at thirty weeks during an emergency cesarean, weighing less than four pounds. Janet struggled to keep her eyes open. Her head felt like a rock she couldn't move. A pair of gloved hands pressed the baby to her left cheek. She felt him, her baby, a wisp of warm skin, and then he was gone.

Just then José arrived in the operating room. A nurse held the newborn up to him and said, "Give your baby a kiss," but José flinched. His baby was completely covered in hair, the skin almost too long for his bones.

The nurses rushed the baby away, placing him in an incubator. A white coat brought out a tube and inserted it into the baby's windpipe, connecting him to a ventilator.

Four days later, Baby Luis was not better. The physicians thought he might have fetal hydrops, a condition that can be fatal, in which fluid builds up in the infant's body. They moved the baby to the neonatal intensive care unit at another hospital. There, the physicians had him tested for HIV. The result, like Janet's, was negative. They tested him for syphilis, toxoplasmosis, and a virus that causes the "slapped cheek" rash. All came back negative.

Frantic, Janet called her mother and sisters in South America. She phoned her father-in-law too. He was a retired doctor; maybe he would have something to say. He did. "It has to be Chagas," he said.

Janet knew about the kissing bug disease. In her hometown in South America, people called the insect vinchuca, and when she was young, she'd wake up with bumps on her body—an allergic reaction to the insects' bites. It was impossible for her mother to keep the kissing bugs out of their house. "If you don't have them, your neighbor has them," she told me. But she talked about kissing bugs the way Americans speak of ticks. They were awful but not a crisis. "You're not alarmed about it because everyone has them."

When her father-in-law said the baby might have the kissing bug disease, Janet hesitated. She thought only adults developed the disease. Her father had been diagnosed when he started having heart problems later in his life, and he was dead now. Her sister had tested positive, too, and she had needed a pacemaker for years, but the device cost $15,000. Who had that kind of money? To Janet, the kissing bug disease happened to grown men and women, not newborns.

Her father-in-law argued that kissing bugs were common where she grew up, and Janet's repeated exposure to them as a child probably meant she had *T. cruzi* in her body and just didn't know that she was infected and had passed the parasite to her baby.

He had a point. While the percentage of children born with the congenital form of the kissing bug disease varies across Latin America between 5 and 10 percent, in one area of Janet's home country, a study estimated that about 7 percent of the babies born there to mothers infected with *T. cruzi* also have the parasite.

Janet was still dubious. She had always been healthy, never even catching colds, and her first pregnancy had been a normal one. How could she have a parasite in her body? Worse, how could she have passed it to her baby? How could she have made him sick?

. . .

When Janet told me that she thought of the kissing bug disease as one that only happened to adults, I realized I had thought the same. Tía Dora had been almost thirty when she first got sick. Neither Janet or I associated the disease with babies or children because the parasite can stay dormant in the body for decades, often up to thirty years. At a conference on tropical medicine, I had heard the Argentinian physician Jaime Altcheh argue that the kissing bug disease should be considered a pediatric illness. "Every adult with Chagas is a child who was not treated," he said.

. . .

In the NICU, so many tubes spiraled around Janet's baby that he looked suspended in a spider's web. A machine made his breathing possible. Somehow, despite weighing only four pounds, he had plenty of hair, as if a thousand black eyelashes covered him.

Every day, Janet spoke to him energetically in Spanish while he slept in the incubator: "You're strong, papito. You have to fight."

Janet always went in first. The visit was forty-five minutes. Then a break. Then it would be José's turn. Junior couldn't go in. She and José took turns walking him around the hospital. Janet didn't know what she ate for lunch or dinner. The hours crowded in her mind and lost all shape. Outside the NICU, she could cry. Inside the NICU, she forced a smile. Everything she felt, her baby would feel. Everything she said, her baby would hear. She told him over and over again, "You have to fight, papito."

At night, when the awful hour came to say goodbye, she crooned to him, "Mami and Papi are leaving now, but the nurses are going to take good care of you."

She turned to the nurse and said in Spanish, "I'm leaving him in your care."

Janet knew the woman did her job well, and she was grateful, but she hoped her words would tap at the woman's heart—that she would take care of Luis as if he were her baby.

More than two weeks passed. The hospital's technicians had found cysts in the placenta filled with multiple unknown micro-organisms, but the tests for leishmaniasis and other diseases came back negative. CDC officials said they would need blood samples from the baby and Janet.

The physicians, meanwhile, studied pictures of the baby's heart. The echocardiogram showed that his right ventricle, which sends blood to the lungs, was smaller than normal. So was the tricuspid valve, which keeps blood in that ventricle from backing up. The doctors continued searching and found more evidence that something had gone wrong during Janet's pregnancy.

Tissue in the baby's heart had died.

...

The day the medical staff collected a blood sample from Janet's baby, Donald Trump put on a tie the color of red carnations and a suit jacket too large for him. It was the Tuesday before Father's Day in 2015, and the day Trump declared his run for the presidency in what later became known as his "Mexicans are rapists" speech.

Trump's words did not offend Janet. She had come to the United States legally. She saw herself and her husband not like the immigrants that Trump warned about in his speech, but rather like the blue-collar white Americans he spoke of—the women and men who were working hard and struggling to make ends meet.

A week after that speech, the results came back from the CDC. Baby Luis had the kissing bug disease. Janet did too. Her toddler tested negative.

...

Stained and magnified a thousand times in a photograph, the *T. cruzi* from Luis's blood sample appeared like the eels with Mohawks, curled alongside violet globes—his blood cells. The parasite had burst from a dying cell in Luis's premature body, and with its flagellum, it was on the move, looking for new cells to invade. The parasite had already reached his heart, where it had destroyed cells in the right ventricle and left behind scar tissue.

The good news was that Baby Luis would not be lost. The parasite had been found. He could be treated. This made him only the second official case on record with the CDC of a baby infected with the kissing bug disease during pregnancy in the United States. Luis had avoided the fate of the lost babies who are never tested and identified.

When the American College of Obstetricians and Gynecologists teamed up in 2008 with the CDC to survey the organization's members about the kissing bug disease, they pointedly asked physicians whether a mother could pass *T. cruzi* on to her baby, regardless of whether she had been infected during the pregnancy or years before. The correct answer is yes, but 84 percent of obstetricians and gynecologists said "I don't know." The survey's authors observed, "The most common response to our survey questions was 'I don't know.'" It was a disturbing outcome considering that almost seven hundred thousand babies are born every year in the United States to mothers from South America, Central America, and Mexico.

In 2006, the federal government convened a panel of experts to establish guidelines for states to screen newborns, and the group recommended that twenty-nine diseases be mandated for screening, including hearing loss, cystic fibrosis, and sickle cell anemia. The kissing bug disease did not make the list, but not because it doesn't occur often. Newborns are screened for fifteen diseases that occur less frequently than the kissing bug disease. Eileen Stillwaggon, an economist at Gettysburg College, and her colleagues found that it is ten times cheaper to screen and treat newborns and their moms for the kissing bug disease than to cover all the costs related to children and their mothers having the disease.

I thought of places like Los Angeles and Miami; Chicago and Houston; the Washington, DC, area and New York City; places where high numbers of Latinx families live. I thought of the less obvious places all over the South like Siler City, a rural town in North Carolina, where 43 percent of people are from Latinx families. How many babies in these places had the kissing bug disease?

One particular group of lost babies stood out to me: the girls. A girl infected with the kissing bug disease, like Janet, can grow up to pass the parasite to her children during pregnancy. In these cases, the parasite does not need the kissing bug. It hijacks the girl's body—she becomes the carrier.

LA DOCTORA

When Janet and I met, it had been only nine months since her baby was born during an emergency C-section. She did not use the baby's name, Luis, instead calling him "the baby" and "my baby," and I found myself doing the same. "The baby. Your baby." The short possessive pronoun and article in front of "baby" felt urgent—a way to pin the premature boy to this world and to Janet.

Every morning that her baby was in the NICU, Janet and her husband rushed to the hospital and stayed there until the sky turned black and waited for news of when he would be treated. It was the summer of 2015. The FDA had not approved benznidazole for use in the United States, so the baby's pediatricians had to secure the drug under specific protocols from the CDC. Finally, the drug did arrive, and the physicians started to treat him.

And Janet? She did not have health insurance through an employer. She was not signed up for Obamacare. She had a green card but had not been in the country for five years, the amount of time needed to qualify for Medicaid. She was able to give birth at the Maryland hospital because most states make an exception to cover the costs of prenatal care and labor and delivery for uninsured mothers who don't qualify for Medicaid.

With health insurance, Janet would have immediately seen an infectious disease specialist who would have contacted the CDC about a course of treatment with benznidazole or nifurtimox. She would have started on medication because while the kissing bug disease in its chronic form cannot be cured, drugs can lower how much of the parasite exists in the body. It would have also helped to prevent her from passing the parasite during a future pregnancy if she and her husband wanted more children. And with health insurance, Janet would have started seeing a cardiologist every year to monitor her heart for symptoms of the parasite's impact.

But she did not have insurance so she and José knew they would pay out of pocket for a consultation. Someone on the hospital's staff gave them a list of infectious disease specialists, and he began calling. One was a wrong number. He called the next one. That physician's office didn't know what Chagas disease was. José was unsure if they understood his accented English. Every phone number on the list left him empty-handed.

Janet said, "Claro, here it must be new and unusual" for the doctors, but she also felt desperate. She wanted to start treatment. She wanted to be healthy. She wanted to be ready for her baby because she was sure, absolutely sure, that he would be coming home with her.

...

I phoned Robert Gilman at the Johns Hopkins Bloomberg School of Public Health. He had been working on infectious diseases and public health for decades in South America, and I wanted to know why so few American doctors knew about the kissing bug disease. He said it was simple. "Thirty years ago when I started practicing in Baltimore, if I saw one Hispanic a month, that was a lot," Dr. Gilman said. "Now it's all Hispanic. The medical schools haven't kept up."

In 1981, when I was six years old and first translating for my auntie about the kissing bug disease, the United States was home to 15 million people from Latin America. By 2015, when Janet's baby was born, that number had reached 57.5 million.

Medical schools in the United States have also lagged behind in teaching about parasites like *T. cruzi*. In the 1970s, Dickson Despommier started teaching a course on parasitic diseases for second-year medical students at Columbia University. He retired in 2009 and started the educational organization he named, with all humor intended, Parasites Without Borders. Most medical schools don't offer a parasitic disease course, Professor Despommier told me. That's partly because medical students won't pursue working on such diseases. They opt for specialties that pay well. "I can't argue with that," he told me. "You paid $240,000 to go through medical school, and now you have to pay that back in ten years. That's a daunting task."

Professor Despommier admitted that he didn't teach about the kissing bug disease in his course. He had about eleven three-hour lectures into which he had to pack all parasitic diseases, and he chose to teach about the kissing bug disease's cousin, sleeping sickness, on account, he said, of the vastness of the African continent and the impact the disease has on the economies there.

. . .

Janet phoned her father-in-law in South America to tell him they had not found a doctor for her. "Come here," he urged. "We'll do the treatment." But Janet was not going to leave her baby, especially not as he began a new regimen of medication.

The pediatricians counted the days. Luis was almost a month old when they started his treatment with benznidazole. Two weeks later, the parasite was still circulating in his body. Three weeks later the first good sign came. The baby's body was free of the parasite. Janet thanked god. She thanked the doctors. She thanked the nurses. She wanted to bring her baby home. They said it would be soon. They said there was no reason her baby shouldn't have a normal life. He had scar tissue on his heart from the parasite, but his heart was otherwise healthy.

...

When Rachel Marcus heard from a fellow cardiologist that a baby had been born with the kissing bug disease in the Washington, DC, area, she immediately offered to help. A cardiologist by training, Dr. Marcus had given up her private practice in 2012 to focus on public health and specifically on patients with the kissing bug disease. Three years later, she had cofounded an advocacy organization called the Latin American Society of Chagas (LASOCHA). Her cofounder, Jenny Sanchez, is a Chagas advocate whose mother was diagnosed with the disease. The two-women operation teamed up with South American embassies in Washington, DC, to screen people for the disease, and eventually Dr. Marcus started a biweekly program, offering testing and cardiac monitoring at health clinics around the city. In 2015, though, she did not have the clinics. Patients knew her as La Doctora. La Doctora would see them at home. La Doctora carried a portable EKG machine. La Doctora didn't charge.

Now there was Janet. Dr. Marcus told the hospital staff that she'd be happy to see her, but they were confident that they could find an infectious disease specialist for Janet. How hard could it be?

Months later, someone from the staff called Dr. Marcus. Janet and her husband had not found a specialist. Maybe it was the language barrier. Maybe it was the lack of health insurance. Fortunately, Dr. Marcus spoke Spanish, and she didn't care about insurance. When José phoned her and asked if they could make an appointment, Dr. Marcus said, "Yes."

Relieved, José asked when. Dr. Marcus suggested Sunday and gave him her home address.

Janet and José had never heard of an American doctor seeing patients in her house, let alone on the weekend. But they wanted to be hopeful.

. . .

When I met Dr. Marcus in a bookstore's coffee shop, I thought she looked like my auntie. She had the same long face, an almost pointy chin. Later, a friend said, "When someone you love dies, you see them everywhere."

With the blaring of an espresso machine behind us, Dr. Marcus spoke quickly and efficiently. She answered my questions, stopped and waited for the next question. She didn't banter or crack jokes. She was the period at the end of a sentence. She was clearly some-one who got things done, who could be counted on, trusted.

Dr. Marcus had not planned to see patients on weekends in her home. When she had decided to work on the kissing bug disease, she actually joined a medical research team in South America and did EKGs and echocardiograms on patients with the disease. She learned to look for patients with bifascicular block—interruptions of the electrical impulses that determine how quickly or slowly the heart beats. A patient with that condition who lives in an area where kissing bugs are common most likely has the disease. Back in the States, word spread about her, and colleagues began consulting with Dr. Marcus. Could she see this patient who had tested positive? The person didn't have insurance. The person spoke only Spanish. Dr. Marcus said, "Yes," and ordered lab work for patients and paid for it out of pocket. She got hold of the medication, benznidazole, through the CDC, and took responsibility for monitoring the patients because adults can have allergic reactions: skin rashes, numbness in the legs, anemia. A doctor is always needed.

Dr. Marcus didn't ask who had health insurance, who was a citizen or not. She saw teenagers and also people in their forties and fifties. She tested to confirm that they did have the disease, and, when they wanted it, she got them medication. One day, her phone rang, and it was Janet's husband.

...

Dr. Marcus's house had wood floors and corners bathed in light. She spoke to Janet and her husband in Spanish, explaining that they would have to screen Janet again for antibodies to the parasite. She'd have to go to a lab.

Janet glanced at José. Their savings had dwindled. José was at the hospital every day, not at work. Still, they would find the money.

José asked, "How much does it cost?"

"Don't worry," Dr. Marcus said. She would pay for it.

After they left the house, Janet said to her husband, "She's an angel."

...

The day I first met Janet, she was taking benznidazole and had no complaints. She was grateful to have the medication here in Maryland but also terrified at the thought of ever having another baby. Even if the medicaton reduced the risk of transmission, which it did, she couldn't bear the thought of having another child infected and in the NICU.

In the middle of our interview, a cry rang from one of the bedrooms in her home. I barely heard it, but Janet jumped to her feet, and I followed her into the bedroom with her toddler, Junior. Toy cars and diapers covered the top of the dresser. A silent television set hung in the corner. Sunshine poured through the windows.

Almost nine months old, Baby Luis had a gorgeous long mop of fine black hair, and when Janet picked him up from his crib, he looked startled, as if he had not considered the room from this perspective before. He glanced at me, then turned to his mother. She called him "Papito" and kissed him over and over again. He giggled. Junior jumped up and down on the bed next to the crib. Janet decided to make fresh juice for the boys and put Baby Luis in my arms.

The baby and I stared at each other. It felt impossible to me that this infant boy had spent months fighting an ancient parasite and had won. He punched the air with his fists and when he opened his mouth, I offered him his lime-green pacifier and he took it.

CANDACE

A few months after meeting Janet and her family, I flew to Houston. My interviews with doctors and other experts had led me to a woman named Candace who had contracted *T. cruzi* from kissing bugs native to Texas. She was one of at least seventy-five people the CDC had identified as having been infected by the insects here in the United States.

The rains were bad that summer. Historic, actually. Seventeen inches of rain belted Houston, and several people died, some of them trapped after steering their trucks into floodwaters. I was nervous about driving a rental car, but when I made my way west and out of the bumper-to-bumper traffic of the city, I found open skies and land so dry it made me think of the desert.

The town where Candace lived surprised me. I figured that if she came into contact with a kissing bug in Texas, her home would probably be in the campo, in a rural area with lots of acres. Instead, the town was tucked between Houston and Austin with ranch-style houses, a golf course, and a historic downtown area that elected officials and business owners had spent the last twenty years trying to revitalize. The rec center offered yoga classes for the town's five thousand residents.

Candace lived down the road from a country club. In her early fifties, she had a slender frame, silver-blonde hair cut into a long bob, and brilliant blue eyes. She met me at the front door with her friend Debbie, who also happened to be a nurse and had been offering Candace moral support since she was first diagnosed. Of course, their friendship stretched beyond illness. The two were part of a competitive barbecue team.

"We're the only all-female barbecue team," Candace said, hopping onto a stool at the island counter in her kitchen. Their team, Smoking Mamas, competed every year at the local fairgrounds, barbecuing brisket and ribs and pork, and, she told me quite proudly, that they had won third place in ribs the year before.

The island counter, long and wide, doubled as a kitchen table, and a candle burned at the center. Candace had brought out a black plastic crate in which she kept binders full of information about the kissing bug disease, but she had a different set of worries at the moment. A grandmother of four, she was looking for work. Her last job had been as a safety coordinator at an oil company. She was a straight shooter, and it was easy to picture her monitoring the hours of drivers, keeping them on task, making sure the trucks were licensed and registered. On breaks, she smoked cigarettes nonstop. "I smoke the cheap stuff," she told me. The day I visited, it was a pack of Golden Bay.

How was she sure she'd been infected in Texas? I asked if she had traveled much growing up. She shook her head. "I'm a poor girl."

Candace told me she had learned about the kissing bug disease in 2014. At the time, she was worried about her mother, who had been diagnosed with leukemia. It felt impossible to Candace that her mother was sick. This was the same woman who had raised four children and worked as a nurse, and, who, a few years before, had paid for a house to be built out in the brush just minutes from here—a home made of pine and cedar and ash wood. Her mother, in other words, was a powerhouse, and now she might die. Candace decided she had to do something.

She woke up one morning, drove to a church that sponsored a blood drive every few months and donated blood in her mother's name. She would make an offering of her body. A few weeks later, though, Candace got a letter in the mail from the American Red Cross saying her donation was positive for antibodies to *Trypanosoma cruzi*.

Candace was terrified. She walked into her mother's house, shaken. Mama looked up. The chemotherapy had slowed her down and the steroids had put weight on her frame so that she couldn't walk well, but she had spent all afternoon researching the kissing bug disease on her iPad, her nursing background helping her make her way through the medical articles. "Don't worry about it," she told Candace. "It sounds worse than it is."

Instead of feeling afraid, Candace's mother thought she should be proud. "You have a rare condition," Mama told her, and she said that doctors in Texas would be able to learn more about the disease from Candace. "You're somebody special," Mama insisted.

As it turned out, the infectious disease specialist Candace saw that week didn't know about the kissing bug disease. He almost sounded enthusiastic when he told her, "I think you may be the only case in the United States!"

Candace thought she hadn't heard him correctly. She wanted to say, "That can't be right." She had read about the kissing bug disease online for two days by then. There were other people with the disease in the country, and there had to be other people, like her, who had contracted it from kissing bugs in the United States.

She tried to shake off her fear. She told herself she wasn't sick. Her heart felt perfectly fine, and the majority of people with the kissing bug disease don't ever experience symptoms. She could be one of the lucky ones. Also, she liked junk food and joked with me that she didn't think the parasite would get her. "My lifestyle will kill me first."

When Candace's infectious disease specialist left the practice and turned her case over to another physician, she pulled her car into the parking lot of the medical center with a certain confidence. She had a rare disease. Doctors would want to talk to her, to know how she felt, what symptoms she was noticing. She marched into the doctor's office ready to talk.

The new specialist explained that they would need more blood tests. The CDC would issue benznidazole under compassionate use protocols but to do that, the CDC had to run its own screening tests. Did she have questions?

Yes, she did. Candace had lived in Texas her whole life. She figured she'd been infected by local insects and that something had to be done. "Shouldn't I tell my neighbors?" she asked the doctor.

He looked at her hard and asked, "Do you know who Typhoid Mary was?"

Candace heard the edge in his voice, and though she couldn't exactly remember the story of Typhoid Mary, she said she did.

The doctor continued, "Well, if you want to be her, tell anyone you want. I wouldn't."

Back in her car, Candace typed "Typhoid Mary" into her smartphone. Up popped the story of Mary Mallon, who, in 1907, was connected to a typhoid outbreak at a Long Island home where she had worked as a cook. Mary turned out to be a healthy carrier—a person who is asymptomatic but infected with a microbe dangerous to others.

I had read about Mary Mallon too. The sanitary engineer who traced the typhoid outbreak in a wealthy family back to Mary didn't like that she refused to provide him with samples of her urine, blood, and feces. He also didn't like that she was single, had a dog, and "walked more like a man than a woman." There was also the issue of her citizenship. Reporters frequently noted in their articles that she was an Irish immigrant. Mary, who could today be called a child migrant, had left Ireland when she was fifteen. She refused to stop working as a cook when public health officials told her she had typhoid, in part because if she didn't work, she didn't eat. She became "Typhoid Mary" in the press, the nickname conflating her with germs. Mary didn't have an infectious disease—she was the disease. The state won the right to lock her up in the name of public health for more than two decades, and Mary died imprisoned in quarantine.

...

Candace drove home from that appointment flushed with embarrassment. She had gone from feeling special to an acute sense of shame. The doctor's voice rang in her head: Do you know who Typhoid Mary was?

She felt like she had done something wrong, like she was wrong.

That night, Candace talked to, as she called him, a "gentleman friend." She was worried about her neighbors. What if they were infected and didn't know it?

Her gentleman friend urged her to follow the doctor's advice. "If you don't," he said, worried himself, "you're going to end up with a brick through your window."

...

Listening to Candace, I remembered how scared my auntie had always been of her friends and neighbors and coworkers finding out that she had the kissing bug disease. We never talked about it, but I understood that she was afraid of becoming a Typhoid Mary, a woman who would be ridiculed or shunned. This was true even though the kissing bug disease is not contagious between people like typhoid or the flu. Most people contract *T. cruzi* by direct contact with the kissing bug's feces. It is akin, in this way, to Lyme disease whereby people contract the bacteria from contact with blacklegged ticks. But Americans know about Lyme. The familiar does not terrify.

Tía Dora saw how Americans reacted in the 1980s to those infected with HIV. The CDC erroneously labeled Haitians a high-risk group, and that community faced discrimination in housing and jobs. Tía also knew about Ryan White, a child with hemophilia A who was infected with HIV by blood transfusions, and she saw the nightly news reports of parents and officials insisting that an HIV-positive child should be kept out of elementary schools. Tía Dora saw how quickly stigma takes hold.

...

A search in PubMed, the medical literature database, confirmed my suspicion: Candace was not the first person in Texas to fall victim to a local kissing bug. In 1954, men cleared miles of mesquite trees and brush in Corpus Christi, Texas. The opossums scattered, and the men built new houses, an entire subdivision. Families moved in, and at night, the opossums, with their long pale snouts, returned to scavenge. No one probably thought anything of it. People had other concerns.

One woman in the neighborhood, a new mom, spent the days thinking about feedings and naps, burps and cries. Her pregnancy had been normal, her baby girl healthy. She and her husband and the baby celebrated their first Christmas that year.

The mother knew about kissing bugs. Most people in Corpus Christi called them bloodsuckers. It was common knowledge that a kissing bug bite resulted in an awful welt. In the spring of 1955, months after the woman had given birth, the kissing bugs became relentless. They crawled on her husband at night and bit him. He jolted awake, turned on the lights, and chased after them, but the insects managed to flee.

Still, the kissing bugs returned. They bit her husband on the arm repeatedly, leaving him with at least one welt that grew bigger than a golf ball. By the time summer arrived with those warmer days favored by kissing bugs, the opossums were battling them too. Someone spotted the insects crawling on the carcass of a dead opossum, the bloodsuckers feasting.

The mother probably did not think of the kissing bugs when her baby, just ten months old, began to run a fever. It persisted longer than a day, so she took her baby to the pediatrician, who found nothing beyond a slightly elevated white blood cell count. Two days later, the baby broke out with a rash on her torso, arms, and legs. Ten days later, she had a slight swelling around one of her eyes. Her white blood cell count shot up. The pediatricians wondered if she had leukemia and decided to look more closely at her blood sample. When they peered into the microscope, they spotted *T. cruzi*. One parasite, caught in a photograph, swung its long body and its flagellum so that it looked like a question mark.

...

Similar to the toddler in Brazil, Berenice, the baby in Corpus Christi survived. Her fever passed. Her heart did not show signs of distress. After all the worry about the parasite, her pediatricians described the case as "somewhat anticlimactic." They treated the girl with an antibiotic because, in 1955, doctors thought it could cure almost everything. Antibiotics, unfortunately, do not work against *T. cruzi*.

If anyone followed up with the mother and her baby in future years, I did not find a record of it in the medical literature. There was also no mention of whether the mother was tested, or the father. The Corpus Christi baby is widely considered the first patient infected by local kissing bugs in the United States since the young Black man from Austin State Hospital was intentionally infected by a researcher.

A year after the baby was diagnosed, a dermatology journal reported that kissing bugs had attacked at least forty-five people in Fort Worth, about six hours north of Corpus Christi. The insects bit people all over the city, in all sorts of homes and at all "economic levels." Back in Corpus Christi, the pediatricians who had diagnosed the baby tested five hundred local children, the majority of whom were from poor Latinx families. Seven children were infected, along with two of their adult family members. The children's parents were farmworkers. The families lived on ranches, and the pediatricians found kissing bugs in their homes.

The more I searched for cases of what I would call "homegrown Chagas" the more I found. Researchers screened Native Americans from the Tohono O'odham tribe in Arizona during the seventies and found people infected with *T. cruzi*. In 1982, kissing bugs in Northern California bit a woman, who ended up with the parasite and a fever. Six of her neighbors had antibodies to the parasite though they were not sick.

A year later, in 1983, an infant in Corpus Christi was admitted to the Driscoll Children's Hospital with a fever. The boy, seven months old, refused to nurse. The fever lasted ten days. A chest X-ray showed that the baby's heart had expanded, an accordion that refused to close. Three days later, his heart had dilated even more. His lungs began to fail. The infant's heart stopped, but the physicians revived him. His pupils reacted—he appeared alert. Then, the baby's heart began to beat erratically. His blood pressure dropped. His heart stopped again. He died at seven months old, though no one could say with certainty what had killed him. The doctors attributed the infant's death to something of "viral origin." The following year, Violette S. Hnilica, a pathologist, examined slides of the baby's heart tissue taken during his autopsy and spotted *T. cruzi*. DNA testing confirmed that it was the parasite.

When Texas health officials arrived at the family's home, in the middle of one of the worst winters the state had seen, more than a year had passed. The officials didn't find any kissing bugs, but they made a lengthy list of all the ways the insects could have sneaked into the house, settled in, and attacked the baby. Holes dotted the walls, and a bird had tucked its nest in the attic (kissing bugs love nests where they can hide during the day). The screen doors didn't fit their frames. Out back, two chickens scratched at the floors of their cages. The rabbit blinked in hers. The kissing bugs could have fed on them.

But the health officials wanted to know if the family had traveled to Mexico.

Perhaps the mother's shoulders stiffened. Her baby was dead, and now health officials poked at her home and wanted to know about Mexico.

Someone said, "No." Maybe she said it. Maybe her husband.

The officials pulled out a display case filled with dead kissing bugs. Did the insects look familiar?

Again, someone said, "No."

A month later, the mother spoke up. She had seen bug bites on her baby before the fever had started. She tested negative for the kissing bug disease. So did her husband, her toddler, and her in-laws. Even the rabbit out back was screened. She, too, turned up negative.

...

Candace did not keep quiet about having the kissing bug disease. By the time we met, she had become a self-appointed spokesperson for those infected. She spoke to newspaper reporters and testified at the FDA as the agency considered approving benznidazole.

"Why did you start talking about it?" I asked.

"I smartened up," she said and nodded toward her friend Debbie, the nurse, across the kitchen's island counter. "Me and Debbie, we talked about it, and I just finally said, 'We need to tell people about this.'"

The two women started with the auxiliary at their local hospital, which Debbie oversaw at the time. The group raises money for scholarships and runs the hospital's gift shop. Candace joined the group because, she said with a laugh, "Debbie kept volunteering me." One week at the auxiliary's meeting, Candace shared her story about the kissing bug disease. Most of the volunteers were well into their sixties.

"How did people react?" I asked.

"Scared," Candace said. They wanted to know what the kissing bugs looked like, and when Candace pulled up photographs on her cell phone, the women cried, "We got those kinds of bugs!"

Candace had never seen the insect that bit her, and she had no memory of a bug bite. No swelling. No fever or rash. But she suspected she was bitten at her parents' house, the new one they had built a few years back. She told me her mother had died of leukemia but her father still lived in the house. I asked if it was close by. She said the house was down the road about seven miles.

...

Candace called her father Daddy, and his house was what I had expected when I thought of kissing bugs—not because it was made completely of wood with a tin roof and looked like the kind of rustic Texas house photographed for HGTV, but rather because the house sat in a patch of undeveloped land. He and Candace's mother had had the land cleared just enough for the house, a cheery stretch of yard, and space in back for the chickens and goats. They had built their home in kissing bug country.

It had been almost two years since the death of Candace's mother, but the front porch still looked the way she had left it, with an heirloom rocking chair and a fine old wooden stove. "It's for decoration," Candace's father told me.

He was a tall man in his midseventies, wearing overalls, and was justifiably proud of all the work he had put into the house. The long picnic table in the kitchen? Made of pine. The bathroom walls? Pine. The master bedroom? Ash wood, but the closet, he pointed out, was constructed from cedar he had brought all the way from Jasper County.

I walked cautiously through the house, then reminded myself that I had nothing to fear. It was the middle of the afternoon, which meant that if a kissing bug was still here, it would be hiding for several more hours. They hate the sun that much.

Candace led me to the guest bedroom, a charming room made of pine with a wide, full-size bed and a vanity table. This was her room when she visited her parents and where she thought the kissing bug must have bitten her. She had come to this conclusion because after she was diagnosed, Candace studied photographs of kissing bugs and looked for them. She searched her house and her yard but never found one. Then the day her mother died, she came to the house to get some memorabilia for the wake. Her father said whatever she was looking for was probably upstairs in the walk-in closet.

She found a wicker basket on the closet floor with a pillow in it. She scooped up the pillow and immediately spotted an insect with six legs. "When I seen it, I knew what it was," she told me. "It was dead. I picked it up."

She had touched it?

Candace joked and said, "Well, what's it gonna do? Give me Chagas?"

It was strange to hear her refer to the kissing bug disease as Chagas. I still associated the name so deeply with Tía Dora and with Spanish, but Candace had the disease and so she had learned how to pronounce the name.

She shipped the dead kissing bug to Dr. Hamer at Texas A&M University in College Station, where the professor and her team inspected it for DNA evidence of *T. cruzi*. The bug Candace sent tested positive.

Her father had not been tested for the disease, but her mother had. The doctors had wanted to rule out the possibility that Candace was infected in utero more than fifty years before. Her mother turned out negative, and standing there in the closet on the second floor of the house, surrounded by pine and ash and cedar, and with the goats and chickens out back, I considered how random this disease could be. Candace's mother had lived in this house for six years and not been infected. Candace slept over for a few nights here and there and had contracted *T. cruzi*.

Now she needed her heart monitored every year. So far, she was not showing any symptoms.

MAIRA

When a cardiologist in Los Angeles put me in touch with one of her patients, she did not mention Wonder Woman, but I thought of the superhero the morning I showed up at Maira's house in Southern California. Her straight black hair pooled around her shoulders, and on the inside of her right wrist, she bore a tattoo of swirls—the symbol of the Akan people in Ghana meaning "Except for god, I fear none." Maira did strike me as fearless. "At six, I was good with a slingshot," she said, matter-of-fact, remembering her childhood in Central America. Back then, when her grandmother's boyfriend grew violent, Maira did not think twice about being a girl in a handmade dress without shoes—she grabbed a broom and started beating the man on the head.

Now in her forties, Maira had a well-stocked kitchen in the San Fernando Valley, and the morning I arrived, she was sporting a pink summer dress with a matching blazer and cream-colored sandals with straps curled around her ankles. She kept her husband and two teenage children on task with house chores—the kitchen counters sparkled. She had worked at Universal Studios since she was sixteen. Her first job was with the cleaning staff, and more than twenty years later, she was an executive assistant to several directors at the theme park. Soon she would be working in the president's office. Every morning, she made sure the directors had their daily schedules printed, and she fielded calls, arranged travel itineraries, and generated reports. She saw these executives as extensions of her own kingdom, or as she told one of them, "When you look bad, I look bad."

Maira was straightforward and unapologetic. The first time we spoke by phone about her having the kissing bug disease, she said, "You get to the point where you're like, if they tell you to drink pee, you'll do it." She had been diagnosed in Los Angeles County in the late nineties, and for years was asymptomatic. Her doctor procured the drug nifurtimox for her. Maira had hoped the drug would reduce the parasite load in her body. In 2015, however, her cardiologist looked at an MRI of Maira's chest and saw that the parasite was beginning to eat away at the wall of her heart.

That was why I was here in her spotless kitchen, sipping a cup of her coffee. Maira had agreed to let me tag along for her annual EKG and echocardiogram. We would see if the parasite had damaged her heart any more in the last year.

Maira had an advantage over the parasite: her cardiologist, Sheba Meymandi, had started the first clinic in the United States devoted to the kissing bug disease and had become an internationally recognized expert on the disease in this country. Granted, the clinic, which opened in 2007, was essentially a one-woman operation in a county hospital in the San Fernando Valley, but it was better than most patients with the disease had in this country. It was better than what Tía Dora had experienced.

California has the highest number of people with the kissing bug disease in the United States—close to seventy-one thousand, all of whom are Latin American immigrants. So Maira was one of thousands in the state who had the disease but one of the few who knew it.

...

From the parking lot, the Olive View-UCLA Medical Center reminded me of a Salvador Dalí painting. The hospital, tucked among the sand-colored hills, had reflecting windows so that at first glance it looked as if the dry land and the bright blue skies were painted onto the hospital itself. The signs hinted at surrealism. An arrow for the outpatient clinic pointed left, almost suggesting that we take a walk in the hills.

I did not tell Maira that it pained me to be at Olive View. I had never brought Tía Dora here, not that it would have made any sense since the parasite was attacking her digestive system and the focus at this clinic was cardiac damage. But still. It would have been reassuring to talk to a doctor who knew the disease, who consulted with experts in South America.

While I didn't bring Tía Dora to Olive View, I did call in the spring of 2010 when she was very sick. I asked an administrator questions about testing for the kissing bug disease, but it wasn't clear what I should do next, and a month later Tía was dead.

Maira had started coming to the clinic in 2008. She had known for almost ten years that she had the disease—a letter had come after she donated blood—but the first specialist she consulted in the late nineties at another medical clinic did not seem to know very much. "I thought: it can't be that bad," she told me. "No one is dying from it."

She didn't know that every year an estimated ten thousand people die from the kissing bug disease, most of them in Latin America. One study in Brazil looked at blood samples from more than 8,000 people who donated blood in São Paulo and followed the donors for close to fourteen years. The researchers found that being infected with *T. cruzi* increased a person's risk of death by two to three times.

The Center of Excellence for Chagas Disease was part of the hospital's cardiac unit on the second floor. We arrived early, around nine in the morning, but patients already filled every chair of the modest waiting room. When a patient's name was called and he got to his feet, Maira turned to me and joked, "You better grab a seat while you can."

Two receptionists scrambled with ringing telephones and intake forms, and Maira told me that they must be new. She didn't know either of them and she'd been coming for a decade. She gave her name and birth date.

"I need your ID," the receptionist said.

Maira pulled out her wallet. "That's the first time they asked me for ID."

"I need you to sign consent forms," the receptionist added, pushing papers over the counter; then she paused. "You have two appointments?"

"I do," Maira said. "An EKG and echo."

The receptionist gave her computer screen another look. "Oh, it's Chagas," she said, as if the disease were as commonly known as the flu. "When you finish with the echo, come back to register for Chagas."

It was strange for me to hear a receptionist reference the disease since I had never been in a medical office where the front desk people knew about it. Tía Dora had been the only patient with the disease at her doctor's office in Jersey. But it made sense. At the time, the Chagas clinic had more than two hundred patients. "Registering for Chagas" meant that Maira was having her blood drawn to check for antibodies to *T. cruzi*.

Writing an observation in my notebook, I glanced down and saw that Maira's pedicure was the color of white lilies. It looked like she was carrying ten white lilies on her toes. The pedicure reminded me that she had a primary care doctor in a swanky part of Los Angeles County, but she had to come to Olive View because this county hospital was the only medical institution in the country with a center dedicated to the kissing bug disease. About 66 percent of the hospital's patients hailed from Latin America, and before the Affordable Care Act became law, two-thirds of the patients at Olive View did not have health insurance. A study published in 2018 looked closely at fifty of Dr. Meymandi's patients with the kissing bug disease—all immigrants from Latin America—and found that more than 63 percent lived in poverty. Almost 80 percent of these patients with the disease had Medicaid or, because of being undocumented, had no health insurance.

...

Maira did not know when the kissing bug bit her. She figured it must have happened in her home in Central America when she was a child. The house consisted of two rooms constructed from natural materials: mud dried in the sun and tree branches. It would have been easy for a kissing bug to crawl through the walls in the evenings.

Maira slept in the house with her baby sister and their grandmother, her uncles, and the man her abuela loved. It was the late seventies. Maira's parents had left for the United States when she was a toddler. She thought of her grandmother as her mother, and in the mornings, the old woman yanked Maira's pin-straight hair into two braids. She tugged so hard that Maira could feel the corners of her eyes pull back. Her hair finished, Maira slipped into a dress her abuela had made and ran with her sister out of the house.

Their lives happened outdoors. The kitchen was outside with the fruit trees, the chickens, and the duck. Behind the house, the black and red beans nestled and multiplied. On laundry days, Maira and her grandmother walked to the river to wash their clothes, and the men took pots to catch crabs.

"I had one doll," she remembered, laughing. "And that was just because I found a head somewhere." She found another doll's body later on and attached it to the first doll's head.

In the mountains, Maira unleashed her slingshot on lizards and birds. When the coffee harvest came, she followed her abuela toward the fields and spent the day picking the coffee beans. A man paid them ten cents for every bucket of beans.

Some days, especially in the early summer months, the rains arrived and made the mountains shake with mudslides. The tree branches rocked back and forth. Maira listened carefully, and like so many children during the late seventies and early eighties, she learned to monitor the mountains. The civil war had begun.

One day when the mountains trembled but the sky stayed clear, Maira, then eight years old, grabbed her sister, and off they raced into the woods. They dashed behind bushes, squeezed between branches, anywhere that the leaves and twigs might cover their faces, their arms and toes and belly buttons.

The forest hid them, but it could do nothing for the inside of Maira's ears. From where she and her sister buried themselves, she heard the screams of women and children as the soldiers plucked boys and girls from their homes, dragged the little ones through the mountains to enact the horrors that would one day appear in newspapers: raping the children, selling them to illegal adoption networks, even raising the children as their own.

In 1981, Maira's parents sent for her and her sister. Maira cried and screamed. She didn't want to go to Los Angeles. She wanted to stay with her maternal grandmother in the home that she knew. But the archbishop in their country had been murdered while presiding over Mass, and by the end of the year, the military would massacre close to a thousand people in El Mozote— half the dead were children.

After walking and riding in cars, and crossing multiple borders with their paternal grandmother and family friends, Maira and her sister reached Los Angeles, where their mother asked, "Are you hungry? Do you want cereal?"

Maira gaped at her mother. She didn't remember her, and she had never heard of cereal. "I ended up eating Froot Loops," she told me. "It's still my favorite."

She learned English quickly, graduated from high school, and around 1997, when she was twenty-four, Maira was ready to marry and start a family. That's when the letter from a blood donation center arrived—she had tested positive for antibodies to *T. cruzi*. She went several times to a specialist her doctor recommended. Then she stopped. The man only wanted to know if she had problems swallowing. Apparently he was thinking about the parasite's attack of the digestive tract. She felt fine and moved on with her life. She married. She had a girl, then a boy. The only time she thought about the kissing bug disease was when she was pregnant with her son, and he came early. She hemorrhaged. The question crossed her mind—could this be the kissing bug disease?—but she told the obstetrician's staff about the diagnosis and no one showed concern.

...

Around the time her son turned six, Maira's heart felt like it was pushing against her rib cage when she took a flight of stairs. "I would panic," she told me. Her heart seemed as if it would burst from her chest. "You feel heaviness, pounding." She was thirty-four, a few years older than my auntie was when she began having symptoms.

Like Tía Dora, Maira never told anyone outside her family about the kissing bug disease. What would she have told them? She didn't know very much. Her husband, Danny, whose family was from Latin America, had also never heard of the disease. So Maira was shocked when Dr. Meymandi at the Chagas clinic said her children should be tested, that she could have passed on the parasite during pregnancy. Fortunately, her children tested negative. So did her mother and her husband.

I asked how her heart felt. Did it bother her?

"Lately I feel like there's air inside my heart," she said. "It feels like there's a bone there trying to crack in two, like it's stuck in there."

In the waiting room, Maira did not look as if she were in any pain. She was joking with me. The first time she had an EKG, she told the technician, "Good luck finding my heart with my boobs."

When Maira's name was called, we learned I could not accompany her into the exam room, but Dr. Meymandi, whom I had interviewed about the kissing bug disease several times the year before, was happy to talk with me. She ushered me into her office, a windowless room with an L-shaped desk and three computer monitors. The short bookcase against the back wall held copies of the *Mayo Clinic Cardiology Review* and a hefty volume whose spine simply read *The Heart*. Gifts from patients crowded the top of the bookcase: a doll in a lab coat, a snow globe. A map of the world hung on the wall. It struck me that if the map were highlighted with Dr. Meymandi's connections, both familial and professional, the lines would stretch from Los Angeles to Latin America, where many of her patients were born, and to Iran, her parents' homeland, and specifically to Tehran, where the doctor briefly went to high school and played on a basketball team.

In her fifties, Dr. Meymandi had a lithe runner's body, and her short brown hair was tucked behind her ears. She didn't have her white coat on, and in a plaid shirt over a long-sleeve top, she could have been mistaken for a high school track coach. I had asked her during an interview once why she had chosen cardiology, and she told me she liked working with her hands. "I like invading the body, closing a hole in the heart," she said. "There's an immediate satisfaction." She appreciated the irony that she had ended up working on a parasitic disease she could not quickly fix in this way.

It is not an exaggeration to say that by 2016, Dr. Meymandi had become the go-to expert in the United States on the kissing bug disease. The few times major media outlets like the *New York Times* or PBS wanted a comment on the illness, reporters called her. She had traveled to Brazil and Spain to speak about the disease, and one time, she received a phone call from Kansas, of all places. A fifteen-year-old had tested positive when she donated blood, and the pediatrician wanted a consultation.

Dr. Meymandi made a point of telling me that everything she knew about the disease came from the work of doctors in South America. She had opened this clinic because patients were showing up with heart failure that didn't make sense. In 2001, at the suggestion of a colleague, she began to consider whether it could be the kissing bug disease, and when they tested their heart failure patients from Latin America, about 5 percent of them were infected. In 2007, she and her colleagues screened patients again. As before, these women and men were from Latin America and already having some form of heart failure. Dr. Meymandi found that close to 14 percent of them had the kissing bug disease. A 2013 study in two New York City hospitals found similar results among cardiac patients from Latin America.

Dr. Meymandi wondered how many people had the disease in Los Angeles County. The cardiac patients at Olive View, after all, already knew something was wrong with their hearts. They were losing their breath or feeling palpitations. It was one thing to screen a group of cardiac patients for the kissing bug disease and another to do so with people whose hearts felt perfectly healthy.

So after their 2007 study, Dr. Meymandi assembled a group of volunteers to draw blood, haul boxes of syringes, fill out questionnaires, and talk with people in Spanish. They went to local churches that hosted ferias de salud, or health fairs, for Latin American immigrant families. They set up tables where people could be screened for cholesterol, diabetes, and the kissing bug disease. Soon Dr. Meymandi hired Salvador Hernández, a young man with a medical degree from Mexico, to coordinate these screenings. He organized churchwomen to act as promotoras de salud, or health promotors. If a patient was positive for the kissing bug disease and didn't want to come for an appointment at Olive View, the health promotoras stepped in to call the patient and talk with them.

Dr. Meymandi and her colleagues tested close to five thousand people in Los Angeles County who were born in Latin America and estimated that more than thirty thousand people in the county have the kissing bug disease.

...

In Dr. Meymandi's office, I asked about Maira. "What will you be looking for with the results of these exams?"

"I'll be looking at what part of the muscle has died."

The chair suddenly felt as if it wouldn't hold me, but I kept my pen moving. I knew that a part of Maira's heart had already suffered damage from the kissing bug disease, and yet she looked so healthy and alive that morning, and she had made me laugh so many times that I had forgotten how bad things might be. I had forgotten about death.

"What part of the heart muscle dies?" I asked.

Dr. Meymandi turned to her three computer monitors and pulled up the echocardiogram of a normal heart belonging to an anonymous patient. The black screen filled with white lines, the valves that keep blood flowing in one direction. Dr. Meymandi pointed at the screen, at the tip of the heart, which to me didn't look any different from the rest of the black screen. "What happens with Chagas is that at the tip you get an out-pocketing. You get a weakness in the wall, and it develops into a little aneurysm."

The language of doctors is generally impersonal—the heart, the ventricles, the valves—which is why I noticed Dr. Meymandi speaking in second person, and I started thinking in terms of *you*: You can lose cells from your heart muscle to the parasite. Your heart can begin to grow a pocket where there should be a sturdy wall of muscle. Your heart can expand like an accordion inside your chest. The parasite can even go after the part of your heart that is most familiar, the bottom tip where the two halves meet, the bottom tip you once drew in elementary school for Valentine's Day. The parasite can make a pocket there called an apical aneurysm. Your heart can lose a sense of time, the left ventricle beating too fast for your own good, and ultimately your heart can stop, your heart can die.

I tried to remember that the numbers are small. Only a few people who are infected with *T. cruzi* and have cardiac damage die from these complications. But I didn't feel any better.

I thought of Maira with a little pocket in her heart. I asked Dr. Meymandi what the medical options were for someone with an aneurysm.

"You can surgically repair it. We tend not to," Dr. Meymandi said.

"Why?"

"When the parasite is there and destroying the heart, we can repair it, and then it's going to come back."

The parasite could return and eat away at your heart muscle again. The parasite could make another pocket. Eventually you would need a defibrillator or, depending on how much of your heart muscle was lost, a machine to pump your heart or, in extreme cases, a new heart, a transplant.

Dr. Meymandi had recently lost a fifty-three-year-old patient to the kissing bug disease. The man was waiting for a heart transplant. "It was pure heart failure," she said, adding that about 7 percent of the Latin American patients with pacemakers in her heart failure clinic had the kissing bug disease.

...

Waiting for Maira that day, I thought about what happens when a disease hides in the body. It is easier to forget a disease that cannot be seen, and a photograph of Maira would not cause anyone to panic. You would simply see a woman in a lovely pink dress with strappy sandals. This is not true for the Zika virus. Dr. Meymandi and I talked about Zika that morning. It was 2016, and social media and news outlets were crowded with pictures of children whose heads had been deformed by the virus. That affliction insisted on being seen.

This, however, is where medicine and science trip into racial politics, raising weighty questions about whom we choose to take care of and when and how and for what reasons. Many diseases do show up in pictures and startle the human imagination, and still Americans don't know about them because they don't affect white middle-class Americans. Consider lymphatic filariasis, a disease caused by worms that nest in the lymphatic system and cause obscene swelling. People can end up with enormous legs or genitals. It is painful to walk. The more common name, elephantiasis, signals the human body disfigured. The World Health Organization estimates that more than 120 million people have the disease, mostly in Southeast Asia and West Africa. Like the kissing bug disease, lymphatic filariasis is considered a neglected tropical disease.

Until I started researching, I did not think about people suffering from a disease that evokes elephants. I did not think about sleeping sickness or leprosy or river blindness. If my auntie had not been diagnosed with the kissing bug disease when I was a child, I would never have learned about any of this. But Tía Dora was diagnosed with this disease and had died and now I sat in a county hospital, taking notes on what a parasite can do to a woman's heart. I found myself wanting to be hopeful too. The rate of people with the kissing bug disease had been on the decline in Latin America. The same was true of lymphatic filariasis. The global health community had started to pay attention. The fact that the World Health Organization had a list of neglected tropical diseases, along with goals for their elimination, was a sign of progress. At least a list existed even if it was one of neglect.

...

When Maira joined us in Dr. Meymandi's office after her echo and EKG, I tried to see her as I had before: the dress, the sandals, the tattoo that told me she feared only god and no one else.

She talked with Dr. Meymandi about a patient support group they wanted to start at Olive View. Maira held her cream-colored handbag in her lap. She looked good, healthy and vibrant. But I felt changed. I was thinking about death. I knew she thought about death too. She had told me, "I leave everything done at the office in case I don't come back tomorrow."

Dr. Meymandi kept refreshing her computer screen, waiting for the echo of Maira's heart. They talked some more. She refreshed again.

I turned to Maira. "Have you seen your heart before?"

"No." She smiled, perhaps a little nervously.

Finally, the images arrived. Dr. Meymandi pointed at the computer screen and announced, "This is your left ventricle."

Maira's heart appeared on the black screen as a series of luminous lines that curved and blinked. Valves struck me as the wrong word to describe the channels for blood moving through the heart. On the computer, they looked like tree branches, waving.

"This is your left side and your right side," Dr. Meymandi said, pointing to black regions bound by the branches. "These are your ventricles." She peered closely at the screen, then turned and beamed at Maira. "I can say this with joy in my heart that it's still very hard to see."

The pocket, the aneurysm, had not grown since the last echocardiogram. The parasite had spared Maira. I forgot myself and cheered. Maira smiled, relieved.

CARLOS

When I first saw Carlos in his Maryland apartment, he reminded me of Tío Papeles. He had ironed his polo shirt, like my tío used to do, and he answered my questions with care, inflecting his words with a certain deference toward me as the journalist, la escritora, speaking overall in measured, soft tones. He was the epitome of politeness, of being educado, as Tía Dora would have said. She would have liked him.

We sat by the window in the one-bedroom apartment Carlos shared with his three brothers. The living room had three twin beds arranged to form a wraparound sofa. The beds were communal. The brothers, who all worked in construction, slept wherever they happened to collapse on a given day. Except for Carlos. He had the bed in the living room behind the television, the one next to the electrical outlet.

Dr. Marcus had connected me with Carlos, and as I sat next to him by the window and turned on the recorder, I felt acutely aware that it was my first time meeting a person who had lost his heart to the kissing bug disease. The parasite had decimated his left ventricle, and so his heart could not get adequate blood to the rest of his body. He was in end-stage heart failure and needed a heart transplant.

Of course, to me, Carlos did not look like a man who was dying. He had black hair and a generous smile. The only unusual feature was that he sat in his own living room with a black messenger bag, its strap across his chest. He called the bag "la máquina," the machine. It was his temporary heart.

The máquina's official name is a left ventricular assist device, or LVAD, and it made it possible for Carlos to be alive. Inside the bag were batteries and a black box that looked like an external hard drive, a kind of minicomputer whose wire entered the wall of his abdomen and connected to a pump near Carlos's heart. This pump did what his heart could no longer do. It sent blood continuously from his left ventricle to his aorta and to the rest of his body.

To stay alive, Carlos had to have the LVAD connected to a power source at all times. Every two and a half hours, he said, he changed out the batteries. When he was not hooked up to batteries, he connected the máquina to an outlet, which was why he had the bed next to the outlet. At night, he plugged in.

When doctors first said he needed the LVAD, his brother, Elias, cried in the hospital room. "Don't worry," Carlos said to him.

"How are you going to live with that machine?" his brother asked mournfully.

Carlos had the same question but said, "I'm going to live a long time," because he didn't want to see Elias so upset and because he didn't want to die.

The black machine in Carlos's hands made it possible for his heart to beat and again I thought of accordions, of the heart expanding and contracting, of a man forced to carry his heart in his hands.

"Hace un ruido tremendo," Carlos told me about the LVAD, referring to how loudly it screeches if it loses power. It had happened one night while he was sleeping. He must have tossed and turned too much and the machine unplugged from the outlet. "The neighbors upstairs heard it," Carlos said.

Another time, he told me, the máquina howled and would not stop. His brothers had to rush him to the hospital. Without the machine, his own heart couldn't keep him alive for long. He didn't know what the problem was, and later I saw that his medical documents referred to a "left ventricular assist device complication."

...

The first time his heart bothered him, Carlos was fifteen. He didn't know it was his heart. He only knew that he needed to cry, and he wanted to be alone, which was strange for him. He had a big family. He loved being around his parents, brothers, and sisters. They lived in a one-room house in a rural area of Central America, a house made of paja, or straw, that gave them shade from the burning sun. His father farmed the fields, and his mother, Mamá Tila, tended the chickens and cleaned and prepared meals and raised the children. The civil war had been underway for five years by then—the death squads and the murders of four Americans including three nuns were known—but that day when Carlos went to be alone by the river, he was not crying about the war.

He had been a happy child, so he wondered why he was so sad all the time, and why his corazón would sometimes beat furiously inside his chest like a trapped bird. He didn't want to tell his mother about his heart or his sadness. There were times when

Mamá Tila would talk to him, but he couldn't focus on what she was saying. She thought he was acting disrespectful. His father noticed too. Carlos didn't want to work in the fields. He wanted to lie down. His father talked to him, and when that didn't work his father beat him. But that didn't work either. His brothers tried reasoning with him. Nothing helped. Carlos went to the river and cried. He thought: this must be adolescence.

And then he started to fall.

He was nineteen and one day, while out on a walk, he fell facedown. His heart pounded inside his rib cage. What was happening to him? Where he lived in Central America, doctors were a luxury. He got to his feet and moved on.

Listening to Carlos, I remembered the familiar exhortation: "Listen to your heart." But no one points out that the heart speaks its own language, possesses its own syntax and vocabulary. Listen to your heart, but who teaches you that the heart cries in alarm by exhausting you, by taxing your lungs, by fatiguing you when you're only a teenage boy?

...

The word Carlos used the most with me was dañado, or damaged. He had heard it from a number of doctors over the course of three decades.

He told me in Spanish, "That's where they detected that my heart was damaged." He was twenty years old and had collapsed in the hospital while visiting his mother. About a year later, the doctor explained that Carlos's heart failure had reached a point where he needed a pacemaker. His first. Two pacemakers and more than twenty years later, he needed the máquina, the LVAD. "The heart was very damaged," he told me. "The pacemaker wasn't helping anymore."

For most of his life, Carlos did not know that he had the kissing bug disease. In 2011, at the age of forty-two, he was on his second pacemaker when he migrated to New Jersey and became a father. A year later, after splitting with his son's mother, he moved to Boston where his brother Elias had found work in a soda factory. There Carlos planned to start his life over after the breakup, but at night when he tried to sleep, he felt like he was underwater, his chest turning into a river and the water rising. He woke up screaming, "I'm drowning! I'm drowning!"

Carlos started to sleep in a chair to avoid the drowning sensation and to avoid waking Elias, who worked a night shift and came home at three in the morning. But a man can sleep sitting up for only so many nights. Carlos finally consented to making a trip to the emergency room at the local hospital. The doctors told him el daño had gone too far. Carlos didn't need another pacemaker—he needed a new heart.

One doctor in Boston grew suspicious about Carlos's heart. He must have thought: Why would an otherwise healthy man in his forties have end-stage heart failure? The doctor happened to know about the kissing bug disease and showed Carlos photos of the triatomine insect, asking if he had ever seen one, maybe when he was a child. Carlos nodded. Of course. He had seen them everywhere back home. "There were a lot of chinches," he told me in his living room by the window, using the nickname for the bug from his country.

Carlos would wake as a child with welts on his arms and legs, the evidence of where kissing bugs had feasted on his body during the night. If he had been treated as a child with one of the two drugs available for the kissing bug disease, he probably would not have needed a heart transplant decades later. In Boston, he said, the doctor told him he had the disease—almost thirty years after he first experienced irregular heartbeats as a boy.

Again I remembered the words of the Argentinian physician Jaime Altcheh: "Every adult with Chagas is a child who was not treated."

In need of a heart transplant and unable to work, Carlos moved to Maryland with Elias. They had two brothers there working in construction. Elias could get a job easily, they thought. The brothers would split the expenses of a one-bedroom apartment and wait for Carlos's new heart. They were sure it would come.

. . .

As we talked, Carlos glanced out the window at the building's parking lot. People arrived, and people left. I remembered sitting with Tía Dora in the hospital when I was twenty-five, the slow crawl of those days. Carlos had tried to get a job at a laundromat, but the manager had wanted to know why he was carrying a black messenger bag. Carlos explained that he had a heart condition. He was willing to do any work: fold laundry, iron pants, sweep the floor. Anything. He was desperate to make some money and to fill his hours with something other than walks around the neighborhood.

The manager shook his head. "What if you have a problem with the machine when you're here at work?" he asked and refused him the job.

The LVAD, the máquina, was saving Carlos's life but making everything else impossible. One time, a neighborhood woman pointed at the bag and asked, "You carry your money in there?"

"No."

"Your papers?"

"No."

"Why are you carrying a bag?" she finally demanded.

The woman probably spoke to him like that because in Latin American neighborhoods in the United States, men do not usually carry bags of any kind. The bolsa, the bag, the máquina, made Carlos stand out. It embarrassed him, and yet what could he do? It was either carry the máquina or collapse and die.

One day, the hospital called Carlos. A heart was on its way, a heart for him. He had to come quickly. Carlos was nervous, excited and terrified, but before the surgery could begin, the new heart died, and he was back on the transplant list.

...

Carlos and I were still sitting by the window when his three brothers tumbled through the front door, laughing and talking. I could imagine the joy their mother, Mamá Tila, would feel to see them if she were here and not in Central America: her boys all grown, one in every decade from twenty-six to forty-three, in jeans and T-shirts covered with neon-yellow construction vests. They halted when they saw me, collapsing into silence and shy grins.

The brothers were a chorus. One told me a piece of the story and another brother jumped in with more. They all wanted to talk to me about Carlos and his heart and the kissing bug disease. It was a family story.

I asked one brother, "Did the insect bite you too?" and the brothers shouted: "All of us!" Only one brother remembered seeing the kissing bug, but the others, like Carlos, recalled the terrible welts on their arms as children when they woke up in the mornings. They had not been tested for the disease except for Elias who turned up negative.

At thirty-five, Elias had a clean-shaven face. He took a seat in the armchair by the television and told me that he worried constantly about Carlos. "It's not easy to be working and thinking what's happening at every moment," he said. "Somehow that's on your mind, and if he calls now, you get nervous."

Jorge, the youngest brother in his twenties, added, "I don't know if he told you. He got lost when he went shopping. He didn't know where he was."

The room fell silent. I looked at Carlos.

"I didn't tell her," he admitted.

The brothers rushed to describe how one day Carlos grew disoriented on his way home, and he didn't know how to reach their apartment. He blamed the disease though memory loss isn't a symptom.

Elias wanted me to know about the medical bills. He picked up a stack next to the television set. "All these are bills! In some way, it worries him . . . so all this in some way gets trapped in his mind, and one way or another, it affects him."

Pedro, the brother with salt-and-pepper hair, said they were making the payments, but the money didn't stretch far enough. Some bills were already with collection agencies.

Carlos grew quieter. It pained him, he told me later, that he couldn't work and earn money and pay his bills. His brothers were attentive. They saw, in that moment, how his face clouded, and they started talking about the new corazón, about what kind of heart Carlos would get when the transplant came. Elias told us he had met a man once who had developed cravings for soda after his transplant. It turned out the donor had a habit of drinking a particular soda every day at the same time. Another brother teased that hopefully Carlos wouldn't get the corazón of a bad man. They couldn't have a bad man, un hombre malo, for a brother.

Carlos laughed. The brothers looked pleased. They had succeeded in pulling his mind away from the medical bills.

...

That day, I did not say anything to Carlos and his brothers about what the parasite can do to a person after a heart transplant. I wasn't sure if they knew, and although I was technically there as a journalist, I couldn't bring myself to ask in case they didn't.

So I did not say that *T. cruzi* has learned to hide in the human body so well that after a heart transplant, the parasite can emerge again and attack the new heart. It sounds like the plot of a science fiction film: a parasite that convinces humanity to keep it alive with a feast of human hearts. One team of CDC experts and infectious disease specialists looked at thirty-one patients with the kissing bug disease who had heart transplants in the United States and found that nineteen of the patients showed evidence of parasitic infection after transplant.

Experts don't know exactly how these infections happen after heart transplantation. There's speculation that the drugs used to keep the body from rejecting a new heart lower a person's immunity, making the parasite's attack possible. At the Albert Einstein College of Medicine in the Bronx, infectious disease specialist Herbert Tanowitz and his colleagues did experiments with mice and found *T. cruzi* in fat tissue. Hiding. "It loves fat. I don't know why, but it does love fat," he told me over the phone.

If Carlos did get a new heart, his doctors would have to monitor him for signs of the parasite's return. The good news was that, if the infection was caught early, doctors could treat it as they would if Carlos had recently been bitten by a kissing bug. The drugs benznidazole or nifurtimox could be used in such cases and were often successful in fighting the parasite.

...

Three months after Carlos and I met in 2016, his phone rang. A new heart was available. Carlos tried not to give in to his excitement. He had been through it once before: the elation, then the devastation when it didn't work out. This time, he called a taxi. He gathered everything related to his máquina: the cables, the extra batteries. He hoped it would work like this: he'd go into the hospital with this máquina and come home with a new heart.

In the taxi, he gave the driver the name of the hospital, and the driver asked, "Vas para una consulta?" You got a doctor's appointment?

"No, it's for a heart transplant," Carlos told him.

"But you're so calm!" the driver stammered.

Carlos was actually scared and knew the terror would get worse if he talked about it. "Tell me about you," he said to the driver. "How much have you made today?" And they went like that to the hospital in Washington, DC, to the possibility of a new heart, talking about dollars and taxis, about what a man's time is worth.

...

Later, the brothers remembered leaving the construction site in a rush and arriving at the hospital to hear the doctor say, in Spanish, that the transplant was "a matter of life and death." They remembered saying goodbye to Carlos. They remembered praying, signing papers as next of kin, and getting cell phone reception in only one spot in that wing of the hospital, under a skylight. They remembered their friends from church gathering at the hospital and praying for Carlos when it seemed that he was having a complication after the surgery. They remembered the doctor saying, "It's a miracle," when he didn't have to open Carlos's chest again, when it looked as if the new heart would take.

And Carlos remembered waking up from the transplant surgery to thoughts about his blue car and his lovely house and telling his sister-in-law Yudith, "I have a car. It's very beautiful." He didn't, of course, own a car. He remembered wondering if the man who had died, the man whose heart was now his corazón, if maybe he'd had a beautiful blue car. He remembered the doctor saying, "Dale salida," let go of those thoughts.

Two weeks after the surgery, Carlos was back home and woke up in the middle of the night on a twin-size bed in the living room, looking for his máquina. Then he remembered: I have a new heart.

...

I drove Carlos to the hospital for a long day of appointments three weeks after he received his new heart. The staff recognized him immediately. "My friend!" the receptionist cried. She didn't speak a word of Spanish, and after a lifetime of interpreting for my parents and aunties, I offered to do it for her and Carlos. It was the usual requests: your identification, your insurance card, your birth date. "I know him, but I have to ask," the receptionist told me. After they were finished with the paperwork, she stopped and beamed at him. "I'm so happy for him," she told me, and I told Carlos, who thanked her.

A man walked by in scrubs, smiling, and called out, "Where's my equipment, Papi?"

Carlos turned to me. I explained in Spanish that he was asking about the LVAD, and Carlos laughed. The man in scrubs turned to me and asked, "You're his wife?"

The question startled me. I looked at Carlos. He was his tidy self in a polo shirt, black slacks, and dress shoes. I was only a few years younger than him, and I supposed I did look like his wife in my pink blouse and dress pants, my hair in a bun at the nape of my neck, my eyes as black as his. I had not told anyone at the hospital that I was a journalist since I figured they would require an annoyed staff person from their public media team to follow my every move. But it had not occurred to me that the hospital staff would mistake me for Carlos's wife, the wife of the man with the new heart, the man with the kissing bug disease.

...

A technician ushered us into a dimly lit exam room, where smooth R&B songs rose from speakers I couldn't see. She handed Carlos a gown and said, "You're going to take off your shirt and put this on with the opening to the front. I'll be back in a minute." Carlos tugged off his polo shirt in such a swift move that the woman shook her head, turned to me, and said, "Men are so fast."

The room hardly had any light, but I could make out a series of scars, of cicatrices, running down Carlos's chest. He pulled on the gown. Then I remembered why I was there. "The open part of the gown goes in front," I told him in Spanish, and he switched it around and lay down on the exam table. The technician told me I could sit behind her.

"Are his scars sensitive?" she asked.

"¿Las cicatrices te duelen?" I asked Carlos. "Se siente sensible?" He said no.

"He should tell me if he feels any soreness," she said.

When she pressed the handheld sensor to Carlos's chest, the monitor next to the exam table lit up with the white tree branches flicking in the wind: the valves of his new heart. A sound burst from the monitor's speakers: a drum. Carlos stared straight ahead. It was his first time hearing his new heart. "The sound is really different," he told me later. His own heart, at the end, had sounded to him like running water.

The technician said, "Have him take a short breath and hold it." Then, she wanted Carlos to put his left hand under his head like a pillow so his ribs would expand. She told me the doctors would be looking for indicators of weakness in the new heart. "If the heart weakens, it's a sign of rejection," she said.

I didn't ask if she was seeing weakness, and maybe she wouldn't have told me, but I don't think I wanted to know in that moment. I wanted only happy news. I had no way of knowing all the good that would come later: Carlos's brother and his wife having a baby, Carlos cradling the pudgy infant in his arms, Carlos's son learning new English words, Carlos returning to work with his brothers a year after his heart transplant, leaving the house at four thirty in the morning to drive to a site in Virginia where he worked on building a tunnel.

Since I didn't know any of that yet, I focused on the music of Carlos's new heart. He did, too, though later he told me that the sound of his new heart made him sad.

"When I heard it," he said, "I thought about the family in mourning." The family who had lost a young man whose heart was now inside Carlos's rib cage, whose heart doctors would hopefully be able to keep free of *T. cruzi*.

CHURCH BASEMENT

One Sunday morning, the same year that Carlos got his new heart, I walked into an evangelical church in the suburbs of Virginia, less than twenty-five miles from the White House. A doctor had told me that after the religious services, parishioners—people like Tía Dora, immigrants mostly from South America—would have a chance to be screened for the kissing bug disease in the church's basement.

Among the parishioners were Javier and Carmiñia. The couple, probably in their forties or early fifties, lived forty minutes from the church but made the long drive every Sunday, they told me. It was their community. They wore modest black pants and shoes, a burgundy blouse for her and a red plaid shirt for him. He had a thick mustache and an almost square face. She was curvaceous with wavy brown hair framing her face.

The couple had met when Carmiñia was raising two toddlers on her own. In his late thirties, Javier decided to become a husband and a father to her young children, while training to work as a plumber and electrician. He had good years and difficult years, but overall, he felt he had done well. Now, sixteen years later, one of their sons was about to graduate from college and the other from high school. Javier had left Catholicism for this evangelical church, and he was happy.

At the end of the religious service, Javier heard the announcement from the podium about the kissing bug disease. A group of public health researchers from a local university would be in the church basement offering to test parishioners. They would also offer free echocardiograms and EKGs.

Javier didn't want to be tested. Yes, his father, now dead, had been diagnosed with the kissing bug disease in South America, and so had his auntie and two uncles. He didn't see the point in a screening—many people, it seemed to him, had the disease, but his body, like his life, was in God's hands.

Carmiñia insisted they get tested. She probably squeezed his forearm, anything to persuade the man she loved. Javier already knew she was infected.

...

The church basement had a central room with walls the color of green olives. A white man was setting up a microphone to give a presentation on pedagogy and religion. Tall and balding, he stood out because everyone else was Latinx, including the men who hauled in coolers of sodas and the women who piled into the kitchen at one end of the basement with bags of fried chicken.

Around this central room, a series of doors opened onto classrooms. One room had a dozen or so red paper dolls pinned to the wall, overlapping to give the impression that they were holding hands. The paper dolls were labeled with the names of children: Simon, Pedro, Andres.

The public health researchers, along with a group of volunteers, debated over how to organize this classroom to test people for the kissing bug disease. They moved boxes of crayons out of the way on one counter and pushed the tables apart to create three testing stations. They hustled around the classroom with boxes of blue gloves and batches of butterfly needles and red biohazard baggies.

It had been about thirty years since Dr. Kirchhoff tested a group of Latin American immigrants in the DC area for the kissing bug disease. Back in the 1980s, he had screened 205 people and found that about 5 percent had the disease. Now, this group of researchers planned to screen more than a thousand people who had grown up in Latin America and lived in the DC area to see how prevalent the infection was.

The researchers had teamed up with Rachel Marcus, the cardiologist who had monitored Janet's treatment and cofounded LASOCHA, the only patient advocacy organization in the United States for the kissing bug disease. Dr. Marcus and her cofounder, Jenny Sanchez, had brought together a group of bilingual volunteers to draw blood and interpret for parishioners.

I was there as a journalist but threw myself in with the volunteers. Boxes of consent forms needed to be opened. A table required moving and chairs too. An office down the hall had to be converted into an exam room. So I helped.

Dr. Marcus, who had worked on public health efforts in several Latin America countries, said, "This is what it feels like in Bolivia. You're in someone's office. There's stuff everywhere." You make it work.

It struck me that testing for diseases is what many of us in the United States have come to expect of medicine and science.

Cures may elude scientists, but tests are routine or are supposed to be. The availability of testing, however, is often less a marker of science than of wealth—a situation that would come to light in 2020 when Covid-19 struck and people struggled to get tested.

In 2016, only certain labs in the United States tested for the antibodies to *T. cruzi*. When the CDC funded the Texas Chagas Task Force with that half-million-dollar grant in 2015, one of the team's first endeavors was to figure out which laboratories in the United States could screen people for the kissing bug disease. But people who are infected—disproportionaly poor immigrants—don't necessarily have the health insurance to consult an infectious disease specialist or to get lab work done.

One physician said to me, "The fastest way to get tested is probably just to donate blood." This only works if a person is donating for the first time. Blood banks do not check repeat donors.

It's also possible to get mixed results from tests for the kissing bug disease. False positives happen. So do false negatives. The CDC considers a person to have the disease if they have tested positive on two out of three antibody tests. But the test results can take weeks and multiple medical appointments. That's a hardship for patients whose employers don't grant them the option to miss work to see the doctor a second or third time.

...

Javier and Carmiñia trotted down the stairs after the church services with a dozen other parishioners and lined up in the classroom. Carmiñia marveled at the rapid tests, which look like pregnancy test sticks. She had never seen one before. Neither had I. It felt surreal that a stick so slender in size could be used to find an ancient parasite. The FDA would approve the first rapid test later that year, so the kits were available in this church basement only because they were being used in research.

How effective are the rapid tests? A few studies in Latin America produced mixed results, but the consensus among public health experts seemed to be that rapid tests served the purpose of screening substantial numbers of people when it was not possible to have traditional tests that require staff to do persistent follow-up weeks after a blood draw.

The first time Carmiñia was tested, she was nineteen and living in South America. "How did they test you?" I asked.

"They used to put the vinchucas on you," she said.

After the acute phase of the infection, doctors can't generally spot *T. cruzi* by observing a blood sample under a microscope. So before it became possible to check for antibodies to the parasite, the primary way to see if a patient was actually in the chronic phase of the disease was to use the method that nature had devised: the kissing bug.

When Carmiñia was nineteen, lab technicians used pincers to place disease-free kissing bugs into a small box. They tied the box to the fleshy part of Carmiñia's upper arm with a handkerchief. The kissing bugs, lab-raised and starved, sensed the heat of her flesh and turned their mouths toward her. One side of the box had only a thin fabric so the insects could plunge their needle-mouths through the barrier and feed on Carmiñia. Weeks later, technicians dissected the insects, looking for evidence of the parasite, and found it. Her mother and brother were also tested, but they were negative.

Almost thirty years had passed since Carmiñia had first tested positive, and she still remembered having to sit still as the insects jabbed their needle-mouths into her skin. "Those bites are worse than a bee's," she told me.

She returned every year to the lab to be tested. The result was the same: positive. After three years, she stopped going. She had no symptoms that she could feel.

Carmiñia wasn't worried about turning up positive on a rapid test. "We're Christians," she told me later. "We say we're in the hands of God."

A researcher pricked Carmiñia's finger and held it over the stick that was the rapid test. Javier stood by, waiting his turn and chatting with other parishioners.

The test stick held a drop of Carmiñia's blood and showed a strong red line. That meant the test was working. A timer went off after ten minutes, and the researcher added a drop of a protein mix. If Carmiñia was infected, the rapid test would show a second red line. The total test time was twenty minutes.

We waited, and the researcher had a long list of questions. Had Carmiñia seen the kissing bugs? Had she lived in the city or in the country as a child? Had she finished high school?

"My grandfather had a ranch," she told us. She was a city girl growing up, but every year, she had spent two, sometimes four months at her abuelo's ranch, sleeping each night in a house made of barro, of mud. The researcher nodded, and I interpreted Carmiñia's answer in my head: a rural house like that with places to hide during the day was ideal for kissing bugs.

We glanced at the white stick. A second red line gleamed. Positive. Carmiñia smiled. She wasn't worried about dying, but she did want the EKG and the echo that Dr. Marcus was offering down the hall.

Nearby Javier boasted to another parishioner that, considering his job back in South America, he probably had the disease. "I was a veterinarian. I traveled all over, sleeping wherever I could. I must have it." He took a seat and held his index finger up to the volunteer. He wasn't afraid of the rapid test. At least not yet.

...

As the day wore on, parishioners lined up in front of the paper dolls taped to the walls. The researchers and volunteers started fourth and fifth testing stations in the corners of the room. The parishioners talked among themselves in Spanish as they waited. They wore their Sunday best: slacks and button-down shirts for the men, skirts for the women. A preteen girl wrapped her long arms around her mother's waist.

As the line of people to be screened grew, I realized that these families—in the basement of an evangelical church in a Virginia suburb—were figuratively and literally underground. White and well-off Americans would not see them, and so these families constituted, in a way, a Second America.

It was a place familiar to me. I spent my childhood without health insurance since my parents earned too much from their factory jobs to qualify for Medicaid. Seeing a doctor was a careful negotiation in our family. We had to consider how much an office visit would cost each time. Starting in fourth grade, I began receiving dental care at clinics for the poor, waiting alongside Latin Americans and African Americans and white Americans. It occurred to me that newly arrived in the United States, Tía Dora would have been wait-ing in a church like this. All the women in my family would have been here. They were part of this Second America too.

...

I joined Javier at a testing station. He told me he had been a rural veterinarian for forty-seven communities back in South America, and he did have the stocky build and serious face of someone who could deal with agricultural animals: vacas, caballos, ovejas. The travel was hard, and like Charles Darwin traversing South America in 1835, Javier had not been choosy about where he stayed the night. "I slept wherever I was." Where he worked was a region of South America that the World Health Organization identified in 2015 as a hot spot for the kissing bug disease, a place where the insects are rampant.

The volunteer at the training station was Jenny, the LASOCHA cofounder whose mother had the disease. Short and petite with bright eyes, Jenny wore a T-shirt and black pants and her long hair pulled into an efficient ponytail. She pricked Javier's index finger for a drop of blood and fired away with the questions from the form. When she asked, "Does anyone have Chagas in your family?" Javier laughed.

"Everyone!" he exclaimed. "My tía, my parents."

His carefree attitude surprised me, but unlike me, Javier had grown up in a community where many people have the disease. It was not rare or strange or frightening.

Later, Javier explained it to me like this: "When you know you have it, you start to save money for the transplant."

It took me a few seconds to understand that he meant a pace-maker, not a heart transplant. It's very rare in his country for people to be able to save money for a transplant.

A pacemaker kept Javier's auntie alive. By the time she reached her seventies, she was living in Virginia and her second pacemaker was giving out. She needed a third one. "The parasite turned her heart into paper," Javier told me. That's how thin her heart muscle was.

While asking Javier questions, Jenny examined the rapid test. Two clear red lines emerged. A positive. Javier had not seen it.

A tall parishioner in a white button-down shirt called out, "Hermano, positive or negative?"

"I don't know," Javier said.

I stared at the rapid test kit in silence. Jenny did too. She looked at Javier and, lowering her voice, said, "The results are positive, but we will take a blood sample to confirm this." It was possible that this was a false positive, but given where he had grown up and the work he had done and the fact that so many of his family members had the disease, this positive result was probably accurate.

The ends of Javier's mouth fell. His face hardened. He did not look at Jenny or me but stared straight ahead into the room with its paper dolls and its chaos of voices from people shuffling to testing stations.

Jenny jumped to her feet. "If you could come over here," she said to Javier, motioning toward the back of the room where a tall man was ready to take a blood sample.

I had watched the blood draws of two women, and it had been difficult. The blood had refused to come, but not so with

Javier. Once the rubber band was bound around his arm, the veins popped into view. The needle entered, and he did not flinch. The blood rushed into the tube.

...

In the makeshift cardiologist's exam room, Carmiñia was already undressed to her waist and on the table and hooked up for the EKG when Dr. Marcus realized the software on the laptop was not working. Fluent in Spanish, she apologized to Carmiñia. Could she and her husband return next Sunday? Yes, they could. In the meantime, the portable echocardiogram machine might work, though it looked, to me, like a bulky Apple laptop from the nineties.

Dr. Marcus squeezed into the few inches of space between the desk and the provisional exam table and pressed the probe for the echocardiogram against Carmiñia's chest. On the computer screen, the valves of her heart appeared—angular and pulsing. Dr. Marcus measured the dimension of her left ventricle. "This tells us if the heart is enlarged," she told me.

Finally, Dr. Marcus said in Spanish, "Señora, your heart is normal. La felicito."

"Gracias," Carmiñia answered, still on her back, smiling as if she knew it could be no other way.

Dr. Marcus wanted to see Carmiñia's heart from another angle and asked her to lie on her left side. "This is looking at how fast the muscle is moving," she told me, watching the screen, and the results were good.

Next, Javier jumped on the table. "Do you smoke?" Dr. Marcus asked. Javier said no. In his younger years, he had run marathons.

On the screen, Dr. Marcus pointed to what she said was called an inverted Mercedes-Benz sign: the pulsing white lines that make up the aortic valve. Dr. Marcus moved the probe around Javier's chest. She had him turn on his side. He was fit, so she didn't have to move past much body fat.

"You're seeing a very normal beating heart here," she told me.

I stared at the screen as if it were a winning lottery ticket. Javier grinned.

Later, he said to me, "We have a saying: 'You'll live until God wants you to.'" He admitted that not everyone thinks as he and Carmiñia do. Another parishioner who found out he had the kissing bug disease that day was shaken. Javier had said to the man, "Tranquilo, hermano. There's no reason to be upset or to be ashamed." But Javier wasn't sure he had convinced him.

THE GREAT EPI DIVIDE

I am a child of the first AIDS generation, and so my friends and I grew up learning about a public health crisis during science class. We were told that pathogens are created equal, that pathogens do not care if we speak Spanish or have citizenship. Pathogens are not racist. They can get us if we are not diligent about our bodies.

Standing in a church basement, watching the line of immigrants to be tested grow longer, I began to consider another narrative because it seemed to me that the kissing bug disease is contained to a Second America, and that, in broad and sweeping ways, this containment is often the goal of public health programs. We do not consistently eradicate infectious diseases—we contain them to communities of color, to the poor, to the homeless, to people in this Second America.

In the eighties and nineties, thanks to activists, AIDS became a public health priority, but the United States did not win the war against the virus. Instead, AIDS has been contained in the Black community. In 2016, the CDC estimated that one in two African American men who have sex with men will be diagnosed with HIV. More than half of all new HIV diagnoses occur in the South, leading health reporter Linda Villarosa and her editors at the *New York Times* to describe it as "America's Hidden H.I.V. Epidemic."

Science does not explain why African American gay and bisexual men are more likely to have HIV than their white counterparts. Viruses, after all, do not target Black communities. One explanation is that in the late 1990s, federal dollars were spent on abstinence-only sex education programs that left young people with little scientific information about their bodies. This policy disproportionately affected Black teenagers. As legal scholar Risha Foulkes has outlined, abstinence-only education programs were concentrated in poor schools that mostly serve Black youth. Zach Parolin, a researcher on poverty and social inequality at Columbia University, found that states with higher numbers of Black families are more likely to spend their welfare dollars on programs promoting marriage between a man and a woman.

Containing diseases to a Second America also explains what happened with tuberculosis. While many of us here in the United States grew up thinking that the disease had been wiped out, we had actually held it in place in other countries. The antibiotics so famously used in the US to battle the airborne bacteria that cause tuberculosis never made it to poor countries in South Asia, Africa, and Latin America in a sustainable way. Now the rate of tuberculosis in the United States is fifteen times higher among immigrants than those born here, and the people with tuberculosis who were born in the United States are more likely to have lived in homeless shelters or prisons.

In 2015, tuberculosis outranked AIDS as the leading killer among infectious diseases around the world, and two years later, New York City had its largest spike in cases in twenty-six years. The borough of Queens—where almost half of the people are immigrants and 56 percent speak a language other than English at home—had the highest rates in the city. The city's health department put the blame squarely on the choices the federal government made about funding. During the Obama administration, federal monies for prevention and treatment of tuberculosis were cut by 65 percent.

Science, of course, plays a role. The bacteria that cause tuberculosis adjusted to antibiotics, resulting in strains resistant to these medications. But this pathogen does not go after people in homeless shelters or in prisons. It does not pick a neighborhood in New York City because people there don't speak English at home. We elected officials who supported building more prisons and who slashed funding for tuberculosis prevention programs, and the disease boomed in these places we neglected.

Four years after I spent that Sunday in a church basement, this Second America made headlines. New York City officials began reporting the death toll from Covid-19, and it turned out that the virus was killing Black and Latinx people in the city at a rate twice as high as whites. Similar reports arrived from other corners of the country. In Louisiana, 70 percent of those who died from Covid-19 were Black though they made up only 33 percent of the state's population, and in Utah, where Latinx women and men constitute 14 percent of the state's population, they accounted for almost 35 percent of the state's Covid-19 cases.

While a number of health officials and politicians cited underlying health conditions to explain why Black and Brown people were maybe more vulnerable to the virus, so many of those conditions could also be linked to longstanding racial disparities in health care. New York City's comptroller found another reason for the higher death toll from Covid-19 among Black and Latinx communities: 75 percent of the people working in the city as grocery clerks and housekeepers and train operators were people of color.

...

In Tracy Kidder's biography of the famed physician Paul Farmer, *Mountains Beyond Mountains,* the doctor points out that there exists a "great epi divide." People on one side of the epidemiological divide, Dr. Farmer argues, will die of diseases related to old age, while those on the other side will die much younger because medicine for treatable diseases is too expensive or the village doesn't have enough food. Or, I would add, because laws put restrictions on who qualifies for Medicaid or who learns about safe sex. Or because prenatal screening tests do not include the kissing bug disease.

The phrase "the great epi divide" makes me think of old paper maps and signs about who is allowed to enter and who has to stay out. It is a phrase that points to an American reality: some people are taken care of and others are not. A choice is made. The "great epi divide" sounds more accurate to me than the more ubiquitous "disparities in health care," which suggests that a terrible thing has happened, but without active participation on anyone's part. Disparities arise. Inequalities exists. These words trouble but, at the same time, offer reprieve: no one is implicated. The same is true of the word "poverty," that knife of an abstraction. A phrase like "diseases of poverty" obscures the degree to which we have made choices about funding for public health.

The great epi divide, on the other hand, says what we have done in the United States to contain infectious diseases to a Second America. We have placed physicians in the position where they have to fight to get their uninsured patients with the kissing bug disease standard treatment for heart failure. We have passed laws so that a mother of two young children like Janet can't get an antiparasitic medication because of her citizenship status or her job situation. We have failed to educate obstetricians and gynecologists about a parasitic disease from Latin America even as more physicians in the United States find themselves caring for expectant moms from this part of the Americas.

None of this is to suggest that we are bad people. When it comes to infectious diseases, many of us are afraid. We don't want to get sick, and we don't want our children or elders to be in any danger either. If that means granting priority to our health over that of others, we do it. We accept the epidemiological divide with the hope that it will keep us safe, and the tyranny of the great epi divide is that for the most part it does shield us from illness. We work remotely and order groceries online to avoid Covid-19. We drink tap water freely without a thought of cholera. When dengue and Zika strike, we cancel trips to Key West and Puerto Rico. Or we travel to Haiti and Brazil and South Florida armed with bug repellent and a rage that is historical because our families live in poor communities and the epi divide is one we have been crossing all our lives.

One morning, I clicked on a *New York Times* story and learned about what I came to call the "epi elite"—families in the United States who can pay between $40,000 and $80,000 a year to have a team of well-connected doctors on call. One of the epi elites is John Battelle, the cofounder of *Wired* magazine. "I feel badly that I have the means to jump the line," he told the paper about his concierge doctor getting a top orthopedic to see his son for a broken bone. "But when you have kids, you jump the line." You jump the epi divide.

I could not argue with Battelle. If I had children and an extra eighty grand a year, I might do the same. I wish I could say that I would place that money toward prevention and treatment programs for neglected diseases, but I can't say it with complete confidence. The epi divide thrives on fear and greed.

The irony is that in certain ways the epi divide does not actually keep us safe. If we live in a region of the country where many people do not have health insurance, we won't be able to get the care we need even if we have coverage. Hospitals close down. Doctors move to towns where they can earn higher salaries. We can find ourselves with health insurance and several college degrees and dragged to the other side of the great epi divide. One study from the pre-Obamacare days uncovered that a woman with health insurance did not get her annual mammogram when she lived in a largely uninsured community, in part perhaps, because the low demand for the screening made it less accessible. Another study revealed that a pregnant woman has more prenatal care services available to her if she lives in a state where the legislature and the governor have expanded Medicaid coverage. More money for health care services brings more doctors, medical programs, and hospitals to a region.

What I appreciated about the image of the great epi divide is that it's not a solid line on a map. It can change according to whom we elect to state legislatures, whom we put in the White

House and on our city councils, and what demands we make of them. It can change if we want it to.

The great epi divide did not change in time for one woman in Texas.

...

At Ben Taub Hospital, the largest safety-net hospital in Houston, Arunima Misra, a cardiologist, fished for a tissue in the pocket of her white coat. She was sure she had one. She knew that her eyes were red and that I was writing this in my notebook, and that she needed the tissue because we were talking about the patient who did not need to die, which is to say that we were talking about the epi divide.

The desk did not have a box of tissues nor anything else: no pens, no notebooks, no calendars. The office itself was the size of a walk-in closet with enough room for the desk, the two chairs, and the two of us. At the door, a single sign read "Cardiology."

Dr. Misra found her tissue crumpled and proceeded to unfold it carefully as if it were an origami crane that could be returned to its original, flat dimensions. She dabbed the corner of her eyes. She forced a smile. She gripped the paper crane and told me about the patient without using the woman's name. There was HIPAA, after all, and also a woman from the press office sitting outside the room. So, I imagined a name. I named the patient Lucia.

The first time Dr. Misra saw Lucia's chart, she thought the woman from Central America had already reached end-stage heart failure. "She had both ventricles that were shot. She had leakages across all over her valves, and she was so congested from back flow that her liver was big, and she was jaundiced," she said.

Lucia was only in her midforties, and she was lucky in one regard. In Connecticut where she had lived, a doctor had diagnosed her with the kissing bug disease. Dr. Misra wasn't familiar with the disease or the parasite, but she knew what to do with a failing heart. She ordered Lucia an ICD: an implantable cardioverter-defibrillator. The procedure requires making a pocket under the chest wall, slipping in a device that looks like a giant silver coin, and wiring that silver coin to the heart. The defibrillator monitors for irregular heartbeats and shocks the heart back to life if the organ stops. Dr. Misra also put Lucia on diuretics and a long list of medicines.

The medical therapies worked. Yes, *T. cruzi* was slowly devouring Lucia's heart, but she was very much alive. And the years inched forward: one, then four, then six years. Lucia took her medicines. She made a home for herself in Texas, after so many years in the Northeast. She welcomed a granddaughter into the world and probably spent hours holding the child and maybe even thought: How could a heart fail in the face of such joy?

Then, in 2015, almost a decade after Dr. Misra first saw her, the defibrillator shocked Lucia's heart one day. The ventricles had been beating wildly, like a bird trying to take flight inside her chest. At the county hospital, she did not care if she was up against an ancient parasite. She told Dr. Misra, "I want to fight." The cardiologist agreed.

Remembering this, Dr. Misra's eyes reddened. She unfolded the paper crane. "What about a heart transplant?" I asked. I was thinking of Carlos.

"She never got funded," Dr. Misra said.

Lucia did not have health insurance, and she did not qualify for Medicaid. She was not signed up for Obamacare, which only went into full effect across the country in 2014, and she was too young for Medicare.

"It underscores a problem that we have in the US and then also worldwide," Dr. Misra said. "I live on this side of the border and you live on that side of the border, so I get health care and you don't."

She was talking about the epi divide, about actual borders but also about the poor people in Houston without health insurance, like Lucia, and those who are undocumented. "We can't save the whole world," she told me. "I understand that too, but somehow there should be a better way."

Lucia spent almost a year in and out of the Houston county hospital. The defibrillator shocked her a few times. At least once, Lucia had to be intubated. She wanted to live, but she was dying, and she did not have the health insurance, or the money, to keep her heart alive.

Finally, Dr. Misra began the painful conversation, the one she has to have with patients who are terminally ill and don't have health insurance. She gives her perspective. Lucia could die here in the hospital attached to tubes, or she could die at home with her daughter and grandchild. "You came here to live with your grandchild," Dr. Misra told her. "Go home and be at peace there."

Lucia agreed, and Dr. Misra turned off the defibrillator. The next time Lucia's heart stopped, she died.

FAMILY HISTORY

I phoned my mother, who was living in South Florida, and asked, "What do you think about getting tested for Chagas?"

"Why?" she asked, alarmed.

I hesitated, then stumbled through my words. "Siblings should get tested," I explained. "When someone's infected, the rest of the family should be tested because maybe they're infected too."

I was so nervous that I didn't explain myself properly. When a person turns out to have the kissing bug disease, they were usually infected at home and all the people who lived in the same house, including siblings, are at risk, too, for having been exposed to the insects.

Mami didn't say anything. I asked, "What do you think?"

She murmured, "We'll see," which was the same phrase she had used when I was eight years old and asked her to buy me a pricey Hello Kitty pencil. It was the phrase Mami used when she wanted to say, "No."

I asked her to put Auntie Biblia on the phone. She was living with my parents in South Florida. "I'll talk about it with the doctor," she promised, and I believed her because in her seventies,

Auntie Biblia had become a zealous patient. A week didn't go by that she didn't put on her sneakers, pack a bottle of water, and take a public bus through the sweltering heat of Hialeah, Florida, to a medical clinic. She outlined her ailments to doctors and nurses and technicians: kidney stones, Bell's palsy, lupus. She complained frequently but showered the office staff with chocolates during the holidays.

A few weeks later, Auntie Biblia told me the doctor had laughed when she asked about the kissing bug disease. He was Latino, maybe Colombian, and he knew about the parasite and the illness. "He said at my age I would have gotten sick already."

That was true. I had not thought about her age or my mother's age. If they were infected, the parasite had spared them. I considered that it wouldn't hurt to get tested myself. I had been in Colombia as a child, and I remembered trips to warmer regions of the country. The likelihood was very low, but possible. Dr. Tanowitz, who had told me that *T. cruzi* "loves fat," had also shared that one of his Chagas patients was a New York City firefighter. It struck the doctor as strange that this man would have the disease. Then, he learned that the man's parents were from South America and had sent him back home as a child in the summers. The doctor figured that either the man had been infected during those vacations or when his mom was pregnant with him.

My doctor in Ohio told me she'd consult with an infectious disease specialist, and after a few calls, I had an appointment with the phlebotomy office where I did my annual blood work. I reminded the phlebotomist, a woman with a blonde ponytail, that I had small veins and she needed to use a thin needle. She told me she'd never heard of this test before. "We had to call the lab." She squinted at the paperwork. "You have a family history," she said.

I opened my mouth to explain that this parasitic disease is not hereditary in the way she was thinking, that I didn't know if my mother was infected, and that I could have been infected as a child from contact with kissing bugs, but that the chances would be slim. Then I closed my mouth. What the woman was saying was probably the most accurate statement about my relationship with this disease: a family history.

Three days later, the results came back. I tested negative.

SOATÁ

When you're the American daughter of immigrant parents, there are certain rules governing travel: You don't fly to the homeland without a tía. You don't take public buses there without a male cousin. You don't get into a car that doesn't belong to your tío or primo.

The rules never felt like rules to me since they had been with me for so long. It was only in 2018 when I boarded a plane in Miami, bound for Bogotá, that I began to feel uneasy, as if I had lost something significant like my wallet or cell phone. I had made two other trips as an adult to Colombia, but this was my first time flying there by myself, and what I had lost was my mother, my tías—the rule that you can only travel to the motherland in the company of the women who raised you.

Everything jumped into sharp focus: the pointy dress shoes of the man across the aisle, the ironed crease of his jeans, the lilt of the Spanish in everyone's mouth, which is so particular to Colombians and which I have never mastered. The woman next to me stuffed her bouquet of factory-made roses under the seat in front of her. She was lugging fake flowers to a country that had sold twenty-four million roses to Walmart for Valentine's Day that year.

239

No one, of course, asked me why I was traveling without an auntie or even my sister. If they had, I would have said that Colombia was battling the kissing bug and I wanted to see what was happening for myself. No, Colombia did not have high rates of the disease compared with other countries in South America, but in 2013, it had become the first country in the world to eradicate another neglected disease: river blindness, or onchocerciasis, a disease I still cannot quite comprehend because it baffles the imagination that a blackfly can bite a person, then transmit a worm that has the capacity to blind its victim. The defeat of river blindness had apparently encouraged Colombia's health ministry, and they had teamed up with the international nonprofit organization Drugs for Neglected Diseases initiative (DNDi) to screen more people for the kissing bug disease and to make it easier for those infected to get treatment.

DNDi had been started in 2003 by physicians from Doctors Without Borders and their colleagues. After Martin Shkreli's declaration that he would snag FDA approval for benznidazole and price a course of treatment at $100,000, DNDi's staff decided to fight back. Along with Doctors Without Borders, they signed an agreement with the Chemo Group (now known as Insud Pharma), a pharmaceutical giant competing with Shkreli's old company. DNDi agreed to provide research support to get the coveted FDA approval of benznidazole, while the pharmaceutical corporation committed to putting profits toward programs that diagnose and treat people with the kissing bug disease.

When I started packing my bags for Colombia, DNDi, Doctors Without Borders, and the Chemo Group had just beat Shkreli's old company, winning FDA approval for benznidazole.

The company later began talks to donate benznidazole to the World Health Organization to treat children who have the kissing bug disease.

I phoned DNDi's communications consultant in Colombia, Elizabeth Pérez, who told me about a project the organization had started in Boyacá with the country's health ministry. The name Boyacá startled me. Ramiriquí, the town where Tía Dora was born and where my mother and, in fact, all of my aunties grew up, was in the state of Boyacá. Elizabeth explained that the new project was located only a few hours from my tía's hometown.

...

In Bogotá, I violated every rule I knew about being an American daughter. I took a taxi to a bus depot in the northern part of the city without a tío. I hopped on a bus without an auntie or a primo. An hour or so later, I landed in Tunja, the capital of Boyacá, and the next day, around five in the morning, before the sun came up, I slipped into the car of a young man named Luis Gabriel, whom I had never met before.

That is not the story I would have told Tía Dora. It's not the story I told my mother later. Instead, I told her about Elizabeth, how she could immediately rattle off a list of zoonotic diseases and what they can do to the body, and how at five in the morning, she looked stylish in her short leather jacket and fitted jeans, while I stumbled along in a boxy rain jacket. I would have told Tía Dora, as I did Mami, that Elizabeth, only in her thirties, had already worked on a Zika campaign in Colombia with UNICEF, and now with DNDi, she was developing an educational graphic novel on the kissing bug disease with the hopes that outreach health workers could use it to teach children and their parents about the disease and the importance of being tested and receiving medical care.

My mother liked everything I told her about Elizabeth. Tía Dora would have too. I added that Elizabeth's brother, Luis Gabriel, was driving us, but I did not mention how fast he drove, how the car took the sharp curves of the mountains hard, me in the copilot seat, all of us practically flying, and how the clouds hung so low that we drove straight into them. When the clouds cleared, I could see a river miles below.

For three hours, we drove north along the Andes in Boyacá, heading roughly in the direction of the border with Venezuela, the weather growing warmer the longer we drove. The scenery remained the same: mountains and clouds and lush green land stretching for miles. I wondered what would happen with this land. The civil war in Colombia, which had raged for more than fifty years, had ended in 2016, at least on paper with a peace treaty, and in the last decade, tourism to the country had increased dramatically. Boyacá with its colonial towns and close proximity to Bogotá offered popular tourist spots. Soatá, where we were headed, was a pit stop on the way to a national park farther north in the country. Still, similar to the United States, the coveted jobs were in major cities, and a Colombian entomologist I had interviewed told me these towns were emptying out. They were mostly home to ancianos, older people, and young children.

Luis Gabriel was probably in his twenties, and he made the sign of the cross every time we drove past a statue of the Virgin Mary on the side of the road. I peppered him with questions about Catholicism and La Virgen del Carmen and his work. He said, "Sí, señora" often, sometimes at the start of a sentence, which reminded me of how Tía Dora had always wanted me, when I was a child, to answer her with "Señora," and I had resented it—why? "Señora" had struck me as silly, as pompous, as unnecessary, as my auntie's way of insisting that I be more of a lady, more like her, that I recognize her as an authority figure, but when Luis Gabriel said it, the phrase sounded lovely, like the start of a poem. By the time we reached Soatá, I realized that maybe Tía Dora had not been trying to make me into a lady. Maybe she had only wanted me to be more Colombian.

. . .

Soatá had a central plaza filled with trees and lined by a string of buildings including the mayor's office, two modest hotels with Wi-Fi, a store stocked with empanadas, and a lounge selling tinto and ice cream sundaes. A commemorative plaque at a corner building announced that Simón Bolívar—who led South America's break from Spain in the early nineteenth century—passed through this town five times and stayed overnight.

The town did not have high rates of the kissing bug disease compared with other rural areas in Colombia—fewer than 4 percent of the seven thousand people living there were infected. The local hospital, however, served the people in neighboring pueblos and those in the mountains, making Soatá a hub in the area for medical care. The pilot project on the kissing bug disease had been underway for more than a year and had changed some of the mechanics for delivering care. It was possible now for primary care doctors at the hospital to diagnose people with the disease, as opposed to sending patients to specialists. The hospital was also stocking the drug nifurtimox rather than having patients wait for it to be shipped from the city.

The day was warm, and the mayor's office arranged to have a local man who knew the roads well drive me, Elizabeth, and two of the town's health outreach workers down the mountain to a vereda, a word I'd never heard before and which literally means a dirt road. In Colombia, it also refers to small agrarian communities, and everyone in Soatá talked of them as if they were mystical lands. They had grown up in a vereda, or they had some claim to land in one. The green onions sold in the market on Saturdays came from the veredas, and so did the giant sacks of criolla potatoes and the enormous piles of strawberries. The only way to reach a vereda was to know someone with a car, or to hitch a ride on the school bus that took children to and from town, or to walk.

The driver, Alberto, turned out to be a hefty man with a reliable pickup truck. He steered slowly down the mountain on a dirt road that at times narrowed so much I had the sensation we were about to drop off the face of the mountain and into the canopy of trees miles below. I focused my attention out the passenger window, where orchids hung like jewels from the mountainside. After a while, we approached a valley. The land unfurled around us. We passed tobacco fields, mango groves, and mandarin, banana, and lime trees. Once in a while, homes with tin roofs and handmade bricks came into view, nestled in that green land.

The health outreach workers were coming to this vereda and others like it every two weeks to check on people with the kissing bug disease. They dropped off educational pamphlets. They inquired about the health of each person they checked on, and noted if the person's insurance had authorized the needed lab tests. They fumigated.

We stopped at a house tucked among lime trees. It reminded me of the childhood home Maira had described to me. There were a series of rooms filled with beds, but family life took place outdoors. The kitchen table was outside with caña brava—thick, long reeds—supporting a tin roof. Tropical fruits scattered on the wooden counter: lemons and limes and an overripe mango.

A boy was watching television in one of the bedrooms and told us that he didn't know when his grandmother would be home. After a moment, we spotted her: Aliz, a woman in her fifties, maybe early sixties, emerging from a crowd of trees, hoisting a pickax on her shoulder. A good straw hat protected her face from the sun. When we sat to talk about the kissing bug disease, I asked if she had any symptoms.

"Yes, fatigue."

"When?"

"Mostly when I walk uphill or when I carry something heavy."

I told her I'd seen her carrying a pickax.

"Eso no es nada," she said, grinning, her square glasses firmly on the bridge of her nose. "For those of us who have to work in the campo, that's nothing."

Aliz used to be able to carry a crate of mangoes out to the road. It was how she and her husband made a living, selling produce to people who then resold it at markets. About five years ago, she had started feeling fatigued. All she knew of the kissing bug disease at that time was that a friend of hers had died from it. He was forty-five. She didn't consider getting tested until three years ago, when she started hearing more about the disease over the radio. She thought: I must have it. As a child, she had seen kissing bugs huddled in the corners of her family's home.

Aliz described to me what Charles Darwin noted in 1835: a kissing bug grows fat after it feeds on a person. "They looked like small balls full of blood because you'd go and smash it and a lot of blood would come out," she told me.

These days she didn't see as many kissing bugs, but they still showed up in her home. Not too long ago, the bugs bit her grandson three nights in a row. He ended up with welts on his back where the insects had bitten him. Fortunately, he tested negative for the disease. Her husband, too, was negative. Both her sisters had the disease, which made me think they had all been infected when they were girls.

The doctors had told Aliz that she already had signs of heart failure. "My heart is moving too slowly," she said. "It's possible that with time, they might have to put in a pacemaker."

She was worried that the pacemaker wouldn't let her work in the fields, and she was waiting for the insurance company to authorize the blood work she needed before the doctor could start her on nifurtimox.

To see a doctor in Soatá, she had to hitch a ride, pay for the travel expense, and lose a day of work. She admitted she had traveled to Bogotá, more than five hours away, and spent a significant chunk of her earnings to see a man who said he was a doctor and sold her pastillas, or pills, for the disease. She showed me a bottle of selenium. She had spent her money on a dietary supplement that had never been proven to work against *T. cruzi*.

Her grandson, around eight years old, tiptoed around us and quietly whispered to Aliz, who startled and asked, "You don't greet the people, m'ijo?"

The question reminded me of Tía Dora's efforts to teach me good manners, of those mornings when I would bounce into our kitchen-garden in Jersey, eight years old, and Tía Dora expected me to greet her with kisses and pronouncements of "Buenos días, señora." I almost opened my mouth to tell Aliz that he was just a boy. He didn't have to talk with us. He didn't have to pretend. The good manners would come later.

Elizabeth rushed to explain that the boy had greeted us when we first reached the house, though I honestly could not remember if he had. "Do not worry," she assured Aliz. "He was very polite. He greeted all of us."

Aliz looked dubious but relented. Her children, all five of them, lived in Bogotá. She had brought this grandson here since otherwise he would be home alone in the city while his parents worked.

Now her grandson wanted a sweet drink. He eyed the mango on the counter.

"No, m'ijo," Aliz said. "I didn't make juice."

...

I spent two days in Soatá, and it surprised me that, as in the United States, both patients and doctors there were only beginning to learn about the kissing bug disease. Local doctors explained that they hadn't learned about it until they completed their "rural," the colloquial term for a program that sends newly graduated medical students to rural areas around the country to serve as doctors for a year. The disease wasn't taught in all medical schools because, as one physician in Soatá told me, "It's not a disease you see nationally."

Elizabeth listed for me the other diseases Colombia was tackling in 2018: dengue, the Zika virus, and chikungunya. Zika had grabbed international headlines, but she pointed out, "There are still children dying from dengue." She understood why pictures of babies with Zika caught the world's imagination. She understood, too, why I was writing about the kissing bug disease. "Until you experience the disease, you don't pay attention to it."

Outside the town's city hall, I met a group of técnicos who had been hunting for kissing bugs that morning after getting a call that the insects had been spotted. The town's pest control team, they had completed an "active search" at a house, lifting up beds and pushing aside picture frames and wall calendars, looking for kissing bugs. They had inspected a dog's bed. Nothing. At a neighbor's house, they did the same. Nothing. But one of the families kept about thirty hens in two coops in the backyard. From those coops, the técnicos had plucked eighty-six kissing bugs.

"Where did you take them?" I asked.

One of the men opened a plastic bag he was carrying. Inside were several jars filled with dozens of kissing bugs. The men had tossed the insects into these clear jars with holes punched into the lids so the insects could be checked later for *T. cruzi*.

I did not flinch or step back or think about bug spray. I had spent a lifetime in terror of this insect, witnessing what it had done to Tía Dora and our family and now other families too, and there I was standing next to a man with almost ninety kissing bugs in a plastic bag. It was so absurd that I peered at the jars and asked if I could see one of the insects.

The technician dug into the bag and pulled out a jar that had a single kissing bug. It was the species *Triatoma dimidiata*, and it was beautiful. The orange stripes at the edge of its abdomen gleamed in the morning light. The more I looked at the insect, the more it struck me as a practice in contrast: the bright stripes alternating with black, the six legs at perfect angles, two dark spots, like teardrops, above its belly.

In Colombia, the insects are called pitos, which is also the word for whistle, perhaps in part because when a kissing bug feeds, it fattens up, taking the shape of an old-fashioned whistle. The woman whose chicken coops had housed all these kissing bugs did not have to worry about eating an infected chicken. Birds are resistant to *T. cruzi*. But the woman was surprised to learn the bugs had made their home so close to hers.

"She said she had never found one," said Johana Cobos Pinzon, the town's veterinarian, who went on the hunt with the técnicos.

"Maybe she didn't see it because the pitos were feeding on the hens and the dog," Juan Carlos Bermudez, a técnico, suggested.

Luis Ladino Martinez had seen worse. Before the town carried out these searches and fumigations, he said, "You used to find three hundred pitos in one house." Still, he preferred working on the kissing bug disease over dengue. "With dengue, it's constant," he said, referring to the monitoring of mosquitoes that required him and the team to spend hours looking for places where water could pool and become breeding grounds for the mosquito species carrying the virus. With the kissing bug, it was easier, he told me. He waited for the call. The work to control the disease "depends on when someone reports the pito," Luis said.

Searching for the kissing bug was his job, and in a strange and very different way, it had become my job too. It was work that felt necessary to me, work that connected me with Tía Dora and the immigrant community that had raised me. It was work that made the world not free of disease, but at least informed. And it was work that kept my grief in its place.

MY OTHER TÍA

Margarita. She was the auntie who stayed in Colombia, the auntie who was diagnosed with the kissing bug disease around 1981 and lived another fifteen years, her heart slowly dying.

I have no memories of this tía. My mother and I stopped traveling to South America after I turned seven. Tía Margarita, then, was the auntie in stories, the auntie who had married my mother's older brother and been very beautiful. Often, I pictured Tía Margarita in Colombia alone at night in an armchair with doilies on the end tables and all the lights turned off—a woman, a mother, trying to bargain with her heart. Tía Margarita sat upright in that armchair. She sat perfectly still. She added a pillow behind her back. She stared straight ahead with eyes half-closed, and she did this because the alternative was worse: if she tried to lie down, her heart would suffocate her. That's what Auntie Biblia said.

It was never clear to me what was true about this other auntie, but when I heard Carlos say that he had felt like he was drowning with his own damaged heart, I realized what had happened to Tía Margarita: her heart, ravaged by *T. cruzi*, couldn't pump the blood that came from her lungs.

What I knew about Tía Margarita's life felt like fiction. Her husband, my Tío Guillermo, was himself a short story. When I was in my early twenties, a few years after Tía Margarita died, an auntie brought Tío Guillermo to New Jersey for a visit. With his generous belly, my Tío plopped into a chair in our kitchen and started telling jokes and spinning stories for anyone who would listen. His stories sounded good. He was the wry observer, the omniscient and trusted narrator. His confidence was staggering. In a foreign country, in another man's house, he sat in that kitchen, not like he owned the place but as if he were truly comfortable and pleased to be there with us, and somehow that pleased us too.

Tía Dora, Auntie Biblia, and my mother scurried around the kitchen that night. They made tinto. They heated arepas and rice and soup. I could not remember having seen the women in my family so animated. This was their big brother and here he was for the first and only time in Jersey.

Tío Guillermo told stories and my father drank and laughed. When Tío Guillermo learned that I was an aspiring writer, he turned to me and said, "¡Anotalo!" Write it down! My father, drunk and delighted finally to have such a man in the house, thought this was the funniest instruction he had ever heard. "Write it down!" he cried, laughing.

My uncle had, at one point, been a bus driver and a taxi driver, and he had brought news from small towns in Boyacá to the state's capital in Tunja, news about men who killed other men, or buses that erupted into flames. The news he brought, like his stories, had the flair of fiction. His marriage sounded like another cuento: Tío Guillermo had loved a woman whose heart turned into a rock inside her chest.

He and Tía Margarita spent their last years together in Tunja, a city only a few hours from Soatá, where I was interviewing patients and doctors. While my uncle had died years after Tía Margarita, their children still lived there, and when I phoned, my cousins insisted that they had a room waiting for me.

...

I arrived in Tunja, and my cousins immediately took charge of my days. The youngest of the six, Juan Carlos, drove me around with his wife and young children to the old colonial towns flourishing as tourist spots. Martha showered me with stories of the city's most infamous woman, Inés de Hinojosa, who in colonial times had allegedly kept multiple lovers, including a woman. Yalile hosted me, turning her daughter's bedroom with its twin-size bed into a guest room for me, and when I asked to see pictures of her mother, she pulled out the photo albums and we huddled together at the dining table in her fifth-floor apartment, her lapdog barking at every passing neighbor.

In pictures, Tía Margarita had a stunning face that made me think of geometry, of exact angles, a face built to clear and demanding specifications. Her cheeks were pale and expansive, her brown eyes deeply set under evenly matched eyebrows. Her jawline was precise, serious, and determined. Tía Margarita, it turned out, had been a child of La Violencia—a ten-year civil war in Colombia that started in the late 1940s between the country's two political parties and led to the murders of more than two hundred thousand people.

"They killed her father during The Violence," Yalile told me.

Tía Margarita survived that war and made her way into a secretarial job at the tax collector's office in Ramiriquí, the town where Tía Dora and my mother were born. Margarita was seventeen years old, and according to my cousin, she worked her way up over the next twenty years until she became the town's tax collector. Soon everyone knew her, including the men with considerable property holdings.

"What she said was law," my prima Martha had told me, and though she had been speaking of her mother's role at home, I wondered if the same might have been true at her job.

Tía Margarita married my uncle, gave birth to five children, and kept her job. In the sixties and seventies, women in general, and especially in small towns in Colombia, did no such thing. But Tía Margarita did, hiring women for childcare and housekeeping. Decades later, my cousin did not resent this. She remembered that she and her siblings were treated by their mother to special lunches and plates of cookies for their birthdays.

The last pregnancy came in 1981. After she gave birth, Tía Margarita developed a cough that grew worse. She had a fatigue she couldn't shake. A doctor explained that it was her heart. She was only in her forties, but her corazón was failing, and so she traveled to Bogotá to see a team of cardiologists. They took X-rays of her chest and saw that her heart had begun to lose its shape. They told her she was infected with *T. cruzi*, but none of her children were tested.

The town of Ramiriquí, where Tía Dora spent the first years of her life and where Tía Margarita lived for so long, was too cold for kissing bugs. After doctors made a list of all the places where Tía Margarita had ever lived or visited, they concluded she had encountered the kissing bug in Villavicencio, where, in recent years, she had spent almost a month.

Villavicencio was some seventy miles south of Bogotá and had a warmer climate. "That could be where Tía Dora got infected too," I said, surprised because my auntie had never speculated to me about where she may have come into contact with a kissing bug and none of the women in my family knew either.

"She would have gone to Villavicencio," Yalile said of Tía Dora. One of our uncles lived there for decades.

Yalile was a very thin and elegant woman with a straight back who kept an immaculate apartment full of gleaming wood furniture. At her dining table, she told me she had been in her early twenties when her mother was diagnosed with the disease. She remembered the doctors saying that no cure existed and that her mother would die in fifteen years. Of course, they did not say it that way, but this was what Yalile remembered, what she held on to. Her mother had a baby boy and a death sentence.

The news devastated Tía Margarita and my uncle, and for more than a decade, she pursued alternative medicine, mostly homeopathic remedies, hoping that she could prove the doctors wrong, that she could stop her heart from unraveling. Sometimes the remedies offered relief. She'd get a bad cramp, and they would ease the pains. But overall her condition worsened.

Still, she didn't stop working. When her youngest—the one the aunties in New Jersey called "el niño"—turned seven, she sent him to live with Yalile so he could have the advantage of a city education. This surprised me. The way Auntie Biblia had told the story, the kissing bug disease had left my cousin, el niño, motherless. But that was not true. Tía Margarita had done what so many women all over the world have done: she sent her child to what she thought was a better school, a school in a place where she did not live.

A decade after receiving her diagnosis, Tía Margarita's symptoms intensified: the sensation of suffocating, the straining to catch her breath. When the doctor took an X-ray of her chest, "you couldn't see her lung," Yalile told me. The heart, so huge, covered the view of her mother's left lung.

Tía Margarita and my uncle moved to Tunja, near their children. As with Tía Dora, the trips to the emergency room grew in number and frequency. Yalile, in her thirties, didn't know what to do. Her mother was dying, but she couldn't think of it that way. No one could.

One night, after midnight, her mother, already hospitalized, began having trouble breathing. Tío Guillermo, asleep at home, didn't hear the phone ring. Yalile got the call but when she arrived the doctors barred her from the room. She could hear her mother say, "I feel like I'm suffocating."

A doctor said, "Tranquila, Margarita. You're going to get through this."

"Don't lie to me," she said.

Yalile tried to barge into the room, but a doctor stopped her again. In the waiting room, she wondered why it was taking her father and her siblings so long to get to the hospital. She watched a man in uniform pushing a portable CPR device down the hall. The man said hello to her. She did not think: that machine is for my mother. She did not think: my mother's heart is dying. All she could think of was that she did not want her mother to be alone, and when would her father and her sisters arrive?

She heard a commotion and ran to her mother's room. Two doctors grabbed her by the shoulders. "Look, calm down. We weren't able to do anything."

"Let me go in," Yalile cried.

"We'll bring her to you. You can't go in."

A nurse called for someone to bring my cousin a glass of water. The doctors dispersed. Yalile sat in the cold chair. She was alone when the door to her mother's room opened. A man pushed out a gurney. On the gurney was a body wrapped from head to toe in blue blankets and bound with what looked like a thin cord. Her mother's body.

Yalile ran to the gurney and screamed, yanking at the cord with her thin hands until it gave way. She tugged at the blanket, unraveling it to find her mother's face—her mother's mouth agape, her eyes painfully open.

"How can you give me my mother like this!" Yalile sobbed. No one answered.

Gently, she pushed her mother's jaw until it closed. She pressed her mother's eyelids down. One slid back open. She tried again to close the eye. She promised her mother that she would take care of her baby boy, el niño, who was already a teenager.

The man insisted he had to transport her mother's body to the morgue. Yalile returned to the waiting room alone. When her father finally arrived, he asked, "And your mother?"

"She's dead," she said. "My mother is dead."

It reminded me of that morning after Tía Dora died, when Auntie Biblia had phoned another uncle in Bogotá, but all she could manage to say was, "Dora se nos fue," she's gone, and I had taken the telephone receiver and said what Yalile had said, "Murió." She's dead. La Tía Dora murió.

...

257

I left Colombia with guilt. My cousin had loved her mother, admired her, and had a good relationship with her. Her grief, her despair, her sobs the night her mother died, and even now so many years later, made sense to me. My sister's grief felt reasonable too. She had been close with Tía Dora, talking with Tía on a daily basis and without complaint. My sister, I reasoned, had a right to cry. I did not.

Before her death, I had thought Tía Dora might change one day. I had thought the years would pinch her corazón and make her accept me as her queer daughter-sobrina. I had put this hope on a shelf inside me somewhere. It was a half-torn seashell, this hope, and I had been ready to pull it down from the shelf, but then Tía Dora died. When I cried, I was not grieving my auntie, but what I had hoped would happen between us one day.

And I had expected that I would change too. That I would learn to quiet my quick temper, to refrain from arguing, to say, "Señora," as if the word were a complete poem. I had hoped, and absolutely expected, that I would be able to practice love so that when Tía Dora's time to pass finally came, I would grieve with a clear and full heart. But that was not what happened.

. . .

Back in the United States, a college student with a tender voice had a question for me.

We were in a classroom at the end of the semester. The room felt too hot. I was perched on a stool at the front of the class. They had read an essay I had written years before Tía Dora died in which I'd described how Tía did not accept me because of her homophobia. Another professor had assigned the essay, and this student with bright eyes wanted to know more about Tía.

"Is your auntie speaking to you now?" the student asked.

All the students, around twenty of them, looked at me and waited. It was a course on LGBT literature. Some of them were queer. Some of them had said so. Some of them had not said so. *Is your auntie speaking to you now?* They wanted a happy ending. They wanted to know it had worked out. They wanted to know it would work out for them too.

"She died," I said.

HER LIFE

I have three dictionaries that belonged to Tía Dora. All together, they total more than four thousand pages. My favorite, the *Pequeño Larousse Ilustrado* from 1987, has five thousand black-and-white illustrations, as well as a color sketch of a man's torso—his large intestine removed and his spleen painted the color of eggplants. On the page that has the definition for tía, there are illustrations of a tiara worn by popes, two tiburones, and the tibia, which is the stronger of the two bones in the lower part of the human leg.

I find this catalog of symbols—a papal tiara, a shark, and a bone that looks like a flute—illustrative of my relationship with Tía Dora.

...

One of the dictionaries is bilingual, and it points out that a colloquial translation for tía in English would be: "a good old woman." It notes that when I want to treat an older woman with respect in Spanish, I should use "doña," which is akin to referring to such a woman as a lady, but if dealing with an older woman who is poor, I can call her tía.

...

The longest of my tía's dictionaries, at more than two thousand pages, is from the Real Academia Española, which officially governs the rules of the Spanish language. It details a dicho, or saying, that when a woman doesn't marry, "she stayed an auntie." Another dicho is "No hay tu tía," which means that you don't have a chance of getting what you want. It's the equivalent of saying, "No hay remedio," which figuratively means that there is no solution, but literally means there's no remedy. The saying "No hay tu tía" is thought to come from Arabic, in which tutía would have referred to a medicinal ointment.

Taken literally, "No hay tu tía" means "Your auntie's not here" or "You don't have your auntie."

...

I have Tía Dora's dictionaries, and I also have her life now. Like her, I am a teacher. I spend hours drafting lesson plans. I give assignments. I grade. I think of my students when I'm not in the classroom and brag about their successes. I buy them sweets for the end of the school year.

Tía taught Spanish to elementary school children, and I teach creative writing to college students, and to me, it is the same work: a study in language, in the way words can pin you to the ground. No hay tu tiá.

One day, dashing up the stairs at work, I noticed I was dressed exactly like Tía Dora: slacks with pockets, a floral blouse, polite shoes. I remembered the idea, the caution, that we become our mothers, and I thought it was strange because I had never intended to work as a teacher, but here I was with a stack of graded papers and a room of students waiting to discuss their writing. I had become my tía, albeit with a genderqueer fiancé at home.

In a few months, I will be buying a new Spanish dictionary, one whose pages are made of stiff cardboard, the kind of dictionary a toddler can throw across the room or try to chew. A dictionary with one word for each letter. Amor. Bebé. Cariño.

I am getting ahead of myself with the dictionary. I should be thinking of baby shower invitations and crafting a basket of diapers and bottles. Still, I return to Tía Dora's dictionary, to the words that will be needed because my sister is giving birth in a few months, and I will be a tía, an auntie, for the first time.

GRATITUDE

More than eighty patients, doctors, and experts granted me interviews for this book, and while I could not include everyone's story, I want to particularly thank the following people who shared with me their experiences and ideas about living with Chagas disease: Graciela Taylor, Sandra Muñoz, María Elena Abrego, Jasmine, Valentina Carrillo, Josie McNeil, Lynn Hodson, Leo, María Elvira Pérez, Jersson Fuentes Pimiento, Clementina Valbuena, and Blanca Mayoly Misse Delgado. The patients whose stories I narrate in this book—Janet, Carlos, Maira and Candace—have my gratitude for granting me so many interviews over the course of several years.

I worked on this book with the generous support of Miami University in Ohio, and its College of Arts and Sciences. The Humanities Center at Miami University sponsored a year-long Altman Fellows Program on Medicine and the Humanities, and this book greatly benefited from my experience as an Altman Faculty Scholar and the time spent in conversation with colleagues and visiting academics. A special thank you to the chairs of the English Department, LuMing Mao and Madelyn Detloff, for believing in this project, as well as my colleagues in the

Creative Writing Program, the English Department, and Latin American, Latino/a, and Caribbean Studies, who make every academic year a pleasure.

A book like this requires much research, and the library staff at Miami University helped me many times with tracking down articles and books. I am thankful to them and also to the library staff at the National History Museum in London and the Moody Medical Library at the University of Texas Medical Branch.

Dr. Peter Hotez's work on neglected diseases and poverty gave me a critical foundation as I worked on this book, and I thank him and the epidemiologist Melissa Nolan Garcia who spotted the editorial potential in my obsession with the newspaper origins of the name "kissing bug" and reached out for a collaboration. I am indebted to Patricia Edmonds at *National Geographic* who heard me talk about Chagas disease and gave me an opportunity to work with her and her talented team. Editors at *Slate*, *The Atlantic*, and *Guernica* also published my articles, permitting me to work with the material I was gathering for this book.

A special thank you to Dr. David Markowitz for sharing his personal memories of his father, Dr. Alfred Markowitz, with me. I wish Tía Dora could have met you.

A very warm thank you to my generous readers: Dr. Rachel Marcus provided insights and crucial feedback. Dr. Louis Kirchhoff spent a vast number of hours discussing *T. cruzi* with me and reading my sentences with great care. Professor José Amador, whose scholarly work on the history of medicine in the Americas I so admire, pointed me in the right direction multiple times. And Reyna Grande asked critical questions and helped me to find the book's final structure.

It's hard for me to imagine this book without the guidance of Stephanie Elizondo Griest and her incredible books of narrative nonfiction. I am also so grateful to Wudan Yan whose fact-checking made this book so much better and to my speaker agent, Jodi Solomon, who makes so much possible.

From the start, I knew this book would find the right editor, and Masie Cochran at Tin House turned out to be that person. Her questions helped me to focus the book, and she provided such necessary organization to the manuscript. Thank you! A special gracias to the entire Tin House team, especially Craig Popelars and Nanci McCloskey, who made the business end of this work effortless; Anne Horowitz and Shasta Clinch, whose copyedits and proofreading taught me so much; Spencer Ruchti, for his excellent fact-checking of the endnotes; and Elizabeth DeMeo, who read the manuscript with such a keen eye.

My friends: Thank you, Catina Bacote, for being the best nonfiction comadre. Pam in Colorado and David in Maine sat with me at the start of this project and gave me the necessary courage to start asking questions. Alice Elliott-Sowaal kept me sane with spiritual sustenance and Minal Hajratwala helped me stay on task in the most gentle of ways. Amy Lewis and Jessie Tannenbaum answered my writerly questions with great patience. Gracias!

My family supported me so generously as I worked on this book. Gracias a mis primas Yalile Sosa y Martha Mercedes Sosa Ruiz por compartir conmigo sus recuerdos de su mamá, y a Juan Carlos Sosa y su esposa, Ginna, por recibirme con tanto cariño en Tunja. Con mucho agradecimiento a mi Tío Ernesto y Tía Magdalena Sosa quienes han sido tan queridos conmigo en mis viajes a Colombia. This book, in particular, would not have been possible without my mother, Alicia Hernández, and my tías, Rosa Sosa and María de Jesus Sosa, whose memories of Tía Dora helped me tremendously. Gracias Mami! Gracias Tía Chuchi! Para mi papi, Ignacio Hernández: otro libro!

While I worked on this book, my sister, Liliana Hernández, collaborated with Dr. Rachel Marcus and Jenny Sanchez to convince Virginia's legislature to officially recognize a Chagas Awareness Day in that state. As always, hermana, I stand in awe of you and your talents. Thanks to you and my brother-in-law, Utsav Chakrabarti, for hosting me during interview trips. On the home front, Zami, my beloved cat, took many naps next to me while I conducted phone interviews. She passed a few months after I finished the first draft of this book. Thank you, my friend.

Frankie Clark heard about kissing bugs on our first date. Five years later, they spent a very long Friday night helping me with research into insect taxonomy. Their love made it possible for me to do this work. Thank you, mi amor.

NOTES

During my research, I relied on these three books about Chagas disease:

Joseph William Bastien, *The Kiss of Death: Chagas' Disease in the Americas* (Salt Lake City: University of Utah Press, 1998).

Jenny Telleria and Michel Tibayrenc, eds., *American Trypanosomiasis, Chagas Disease: One Hundred Years of Research*, 2nd ed. (New York: Elsevier, 2017).

Rodrigo Zeledón et al., *An Appraisal of the Status of Chagas Disease in the United States* (New York: Elsevier, 2012).

A WORD SHE WHISPERS

Much of the information about Chagas disease in this chapter is drawn from two sources: Caryn Bern, "Chagas' Disease," *New England Journal of Medicine* 373, no. 5 (July 2015): 456–66, and Maria Carmo Pereira Nunes et al., "Chagas Cardiomyopathy: An Update of Current Clinical Knowledge and Management: A Scientific Statement from the American Heart Association," *Circulation* 138, no. 12 (September 2018): e169–e209.

PAGE 2 *Few people, though, are diagnosed and fewer receive treatment:* Jennifer Manne-Goehler, Michael R. Reich, and Veronika J. Wirtz, "Access to Care for Chagas Disease in the United States: A Health Systems Analysis," *American Journal of Tropical Medicine and Hygiene* 93, no. 1 (July 2015): 108–113.

PAGE 2 *It belts out the familiar tune:* Fay Bound Alberti, *Matters of the Heart: History, Medicine, and Emotion* (Oxford: Oxford University Press, 2010), 62.

PAGE 2 *In 1836, Dr. Peter Mere Latham insisted:* W. B. Fye, "Pierre Mere Latham, 1789–1875," *Clinical Cardiology* 12, no. 10 (October 1989): 609–11.

PAGE 3 *They are, like Tía Dora, immigrants:* Susan P. Montgomery et al., "Neglected Parasitic Infections in the United States: Chagas Disease," *American Journal of Tropical Medicine and Hygiene* 90, no. 5 (May 2014): 814–18.

PAGE 3 *Close to six million people are currently infected:* World Health Organization, "Chagas Disease in Latin America: An Epidemiological Update Based on 2010 Estimates," *Weekly Epidemiological Record* 90, no. 6 (2015): 33–43.

PAGE 3 *Every year, more than ten thousand people die:* "Chagas Disease (American Trypanosomiasis)," World Health Organization, https://www.who.int/chagas/epidemiology/en/.

PAGE 3 *In the United States, women are not routinely screened:* Montgomery, "Neglected Parasitic Infections," 814–18.

PAGE 3 *My auntie also did not know that blood banks:* US Food and Drug Administration, *Use of Serological Tests to Reduce the Risk of Transmission of Trypanosoma cruzi Infection in Blood and Blood Components* (Silver Spring, MD: Office of Communication, Outreach and Development, 2017).

PAGE 3 *The World Health Organziation classifies it:* David H Molyneux, Lorenzo Savioli, and Dirk Engels, "Neglected Tropical Diseases: Progress Towards Addressing the Chronic Pandemic," *Lancet* 389, no. 10066 (January 2017): 312–25.

NOTES

PAGE 4 The New Yorker *has called the kissing bug disease:* Jennie Erin Smith, "America's War on the Kissing Bug," *The New Yorker,* November 20, 2015.

PALABRAS

PAGE 7 *In the seventies, Colombia's civil war remained tucked away:* Catherine C. LeGrand, "The Colombian Crisis in Historical Perspective," *Canadian Journal of Latin American and Caribbean Studies* 28, no. 55/56 (2003): 165–209.

PAGE 7 *Airplanes flew from Bogotá without exploding:* "All 107 Aboard Killed as Colombian Jet Explodes," *New York Times,* November 28, 1989. For a compelling novelist's interpretation of Colombia during the 1980s, I recommend Juan Gabriel Vásquez, *The Sound of Things Falling* (New York: Riverhead, 2014).

PAGE 7 *no one worried about being kidnapped:* Sibylla Brodzinsky, "Kidnapping in Colombia: The Role of Abductions in Decades-Long Conflict," *Christian Science Monitor,* June 21, 2013. For a poignant fictional account of the kidnappings, I recommend Ingrid Rojas Contreras, *Fruit of the Drunken Tree* (New York: Doubleday, 2018).

PAGE 7 *At the Palace of Justice, the Supreme Court judges:* Ana Carrigan, *The Palace of Justice: A Colombian Tragedy* (New York: Four Walls Eight Windows, 1993); and Joe Parkin Daniels, "Colombia Remembers One of the Bloodiest Events of Its Long Conflict," VICE, November 7, 2015.

PAGE 12 *My auntie's large intestine had dilated:* Fritz Köberle, "Chagas' Disease and Chagas' Syndromes: The Pathology of American Trypanosomiasis," *Advances in Parasitology* 6 (1968): 63–116.

PAGE 15 *In an article in* the New York Times, *years after his death:* Barron H. Lerner, "Young Doctors Learn Quickly In the Hot Seat," *New York Times,* March 14, 2006.

NOTES

PAGE 15 *This may explain how Dr. Markowitz diagnosed Tía Dora:* Köberle, "Chagas' Disease and Chagas' Syndromes" 63–116.

PAGE 15 *A man can, as Tía Dora did, appear pregnant:* Joseph William Bastien, *The Kiss of Death: Chagas' Disease in the Americas* (Salt Lake City: University of Utah Press, 1998), 21.

THE APPLE

PAGE 20 *The son of Jewish immigrants, Dr. Markowitz apparently knew as much:* Dr. David Markowitz (Dr. Alfred Markowitz's son) in discussion with the author, May 17, 2019.

PAGE 21 *outside of Miami, our town had the most Cubans:* Jesus Rangel, "A Touch of Havana Brings Life to Union City," *New York Times*, February 22, 1988.

BICHOS

PAGE 27 *The fruit was contaminated by a bicho:* The parasite that causes the kissing bug disease can be contracted through what is called "oral transmission," which means the parasite is in food or drink and ingested. Belkisyolé Alarcón de Noya et al., "Update on Oral Chagas Disease Outbreaks in Venezuela: Epidemiological, Clinical and Diagnostic Approaches," *Memórias do Instituto Oswaldo Cruz* 110, no. 3 (May 2015): 377–86.

PAGE 31 *In March 1835, he and his guide rode mules:* Charles Darwin, *The Voyage of the Beagle*, ed. Leonard Engel (New York: Anchor Books, 1962), 331.

PAGE 32 *when they finally escaped the locusts and reached Luján de Cuyo:* Darwin seems to have mistakenly identified Luján de Cuyo as Luxan in his writings. "Breve historia de nuestro querido Luján de Cuyo," Noticias Lujaninas Diario Online, May 11, 2019.

PAGE 32 *he wrote how "disgusting" it was to feel:* R.D. Keynes, *Charles Darwin's Beagle Dairy,* (Cambridge University Press, 2001), 315.

PAGE 32 *In 1959, nearly eight decades after his death:* Saul Adler, "Darwin's Illness," *Nature* 184, no. 4693 (October 1959): 1102–3; and A. W. Woodruff, "Darwin's Health in Relation to His Voyage to South America," *British Medical Journal* 1, no. 5437 (March 1965): 745–50.

PAGE 32 *He was certainly sick for most of his life:* Anthony K. Campbell and Stephanie B. Matthews, "Darwin Diagnosed?" *Biological Journal of the Linnean Society* 116, no. 4 (December 2015): 964–84.

PAGE 32 *The only fact we know for sure from Darwin's notebooks:* Darwin collected a kissing bug from Iquique which at the time belonged to Peru but is now considered part of Chile. Kenneth G. V. Smith, "Darwin's Insects," 89 and 96–97.

PAGE 33 *In Chile, the kissing bug was "flat as a wafer":* Darwin, *The Voyage of the Beagle,* 331. Details of the officer being bitten are also from this source.

PAGE 33 *Eighteen days later, it wanted to feed again:* Smith, "Darwin's Insects," 96.

PAGE 33 *In the 1500s, three hundred years before Darwin traveled:* Felipe Guhl, "Chagas Disease in Pre-Colombian Civilizations," in *American Trypanosomiasis, Chagas Disease: One Hundred Years of Research,* 2nd eds., ed. Jenny Telleria and Michel Tibayrenc (New York: Elsevier, 2017), 33.

PAGE 33 *In 1855, twenty years after Charles Darwin encountered the kissing bugs:* Arthur V. Evans and James N. Hogue, *Introduction to California Beetles* (Berkeley: University of California Press, 2004), 12.

PAGE 33 *He named it* Conorhinus sanguisuga: John Le Conte and A. Retzius, "September 25th; Descriptions of New Species of Astacus from Georgia; On a New Species of Gelasimus; Remarks on Two Species of American Cimex; On Artificially Formed Skulls from the Ancient World," *Proceedings of the Academy of Natural Sciences of Philadelphia* 7 (1854): 399–408.

PAGE 34 *Kissing bugs came to be called triatomine insects:* M.D. Bargues, C. Schofield, and J.-P. Dujardin. "Classification and Systematics of the Triatominae," in *American Trypanosomiasis, Chagas Disease: One Hundred Years of Research*, 2nd ed., eds. Jenny Telleria and Michel Tibayrenc. (New York: Elsevier, 2017).

PAGE 34 *All over the Americas, though, people adopted other names:* Guhl, "Chagas Disease in Pre-Colombian Civilizations," 31–32.

PAGE 34 *In Texas and the Southwest, people have called the kissing bug a bloodsucker:* Norman C. Woody and Hannah B. Woody, "American Trypanosomiasis (Chagas' Disease); First Indigenous Case in the United States," *Journal of the American Medical Association* 159, no. 7 (October 15, 1955): 676–677.

PAGE 34 *Vinchuca means "bug that lets itself fall":* Guhl, "Chagas Disease in Pre-Colombian Civilizations," 30.

PAGE 35 *It began when when an elderly man woke up:* "Bite of a Strange Bug," *Washington Post*, June 20, 1899; and Melissa Nolan Garcia et al., "The 1899 United States Kissing Bug Epidemic," *PLOS Neglected Tropical Diseases* 9, no. 12 (December 2015).

PAGE 35 *"In the absence of a scientific name for the creature":* "An Entomological Mystery," *Washington Post*, June 23, 1899.

PAGE 35 *In New York City, Bellevue Hospital admitted six people:* "More 'Kissing Bug' Victims," *New York Times*, July 2, 1899.

PAGE 35 *Boston alone had a dozen cases:* "Twelve Kissing Bug Victims," *Boston Daily Globe*, July 25, 1899.

PAGE 35 *One Delaware newspaper reported that kissing bugs:* "Kissing Bug Is Here," *Wilmington Daily Republican,* June 30, 1899.

PAGE 35 *In Washington, DC, men with bandaged faces:* L. O. Howard, "Spider Bites and 'Kissing Bugs,'" *Popular Science Monthly* 56 (November 1899): 31–41.

PAGE 36 *Newspapers named the mysterious insect the kissing bug:* "'Kissing Bugs' at Work," *New York Times,* June 29, 1899.

PAGE 36 *In Philadelphia, a six-year-old boy woke on a Tuesday morning:* "Fatal Bite of Kissing Bug," *Boston Daily Globe,* July 6, 1899.

PAGE 36 *A two-year-old girl died in Trenton:* "Kissing Bug's Bite Fatal," *Washington Post,* July 10, 1899.

PAGE 36 *In Chicago, a doctor wrote "kissing bug":* "Killed by Kissing Bug," *Chicago Daily Tribune,* July 19, 1899.

PAGE 36 *Warnings about kissing bugs appeared in newspapers:* "The Kissing Bug in El Paso," *El Paso Daily Herald,* July 13, 1899; and "The Kissing Bug," *Las Vegas Daily Optic,* July 12, 1899.

PAGE 36 *One entomologist insisted that the insect bit people on the mouth:* "A Kissing Bug Theory," *Chicago Daily Tribune,* July 13, 1899.

PAGE 36 *A doctor proposed that it was probably a "nervous disorder":* "Criminal Unmasked," *Evening Star,* June 23, 1899.

PAGE 37 *The giant, swollen lips, he wrote, were due:* John S. Blankman, letter to the editor, *Evening Star,* June 23, 1899.

PAGE 37 *Shopkeepers sold kissing bug jewelry:* Irene Rowland, "Lady and the Beetle," *Washington Post,* July 16, 1899.

PAGE 37 *Poets wrote lyrical odes to the insect:* Robert E. Bartholomew and Hilary Evans, *Panic Attacks: Media Manipulation and Mass Delusion* (Stroud, Gloucestershire: Sutton Publishing, 2004).

PAGE 37 *The* Chicago Daily Tribune *ran a story:* "Yankee Kissing Bug a Terror," *Chicago Daily Tribune*, September 3, 1899.

PAGE 37 *Leland Ossian Howard, the head of entomology at the US Department of Agriculture:* Howard, "Spider Bites and 'Kissing Bugs,'" 31–41.

PAGE 37 *They turned to their archives:* "'Kissing Bug' Accused," *New York Times*, August 26, 1939.

DR. CHAGAS

I found these five sources particularly helpful for details about the life and work of Dr. Carlos Chagas:

Tania C. de Araujo-Jorge, Jenny Telleria, and Jaime Rios-Dalenz, "History of the Discovery of the *American Trypanosomiasis (Chagas Disease),*" in *American Trypanosomiasis, Chagas Disease: One Hundred Years of Research*, 2nd ed., eds. Jenny Telleria and Michel Tibayrenc (New York: Elsevier, 2017), 1–18.

Carlos Chagas, "The Discovery of *Trypanosoma cruzi* and of American Trypanosomiasis: Historic Retrospect," *Memórias do Instituto Oswaldo Cruz* 15, no. 1 (1922): 3–11.

Simone Petraglia Kropf and Magali Romero Sá, "The Discovery of *Trypanosoma cruzi* and Chagas Disease (1908–1909): Tropical Medicine in Brazil," *História, Ciências, Saúde-Manguinhos* 16, suppl. 1 (July 2009): 13–34.

Jonathan Leonard, "Carlos Chagas: Pionero de la Salud en el Interior del Brasil," *Boletín de la Oficina Sanitaria Panamericana* 110, no. 3 (March 1991): 185–198.

Nancy Leys Stepan, "Appearances and Disappearances," chap. 6 in *Picturing Tropical Nature* (Ithaca: Cornell University Press, 2001).

PAGE 40 *Building an empire meant encountering pathogens:* For a helpful overview about the rise of "tropical medicine," I recommend John Farley, *Bilharzia: A History of Imperial Tropical Medicine* (Cambridge: Cambridge University Press, 1991).

PAGE 41 *By the 1890s, though, they had embraced germ theory:* Frank Snowden, "Epidemics in Western Society Since 1600" (Yale University: Open Yale Courses), http://oyc.yale.edu. License: Creative Commons BY-NC-SA.

PAGE 41 *No one knew at the time that kissing bugs were guilty:* Philippe Büscher et al., "Human African Trypanosomiasis," *Lancet* 390, no. 10110 (June 2017): 2397–2409.

PAGE 41 *The disease killed more than a quarter of a million people:* For this and other historical details about the disease, see Maryinez Lyons, *The Colonial Disease: A Social History of Sleeping Sickness in Northern Zaire, 1900–1940* (Cambridge: Cambridge University Press, 1992).

PAGE 42 *By the start of the twentieth century, Brazil:* José Amador, *Medicine and Nation Building in the Americas, 1890–1940* (Nashville: Vanderbilt University Press, 2015); and Stepan, "Appearances and Disappearances," chap. 6 in *Picturing Tropical Nature.*

PAGE 43 *The new buildings gleamed in the sunlight:* Teresa Meade, "'Civilizing Rio de Janeiro': The Public Health Campaign and the Riot of 1904," *Journal of Social History* 20, no. 2 (Winter 1986): 301–22. Other details about the yellow fever campaign are from this article.

PAGE 46 *In the 1940s, Dr. Salvador Mazza was able to find:* Juan Pablo Zabala, "Historia de la enfermedad de Chagas en Argentina: evolución conceptual, institucional y política," *História, Ciências, Saúde-Manguinhos* 16, suppl. 1 (July 2009): 62.

PAGE 47 *By 1985, more than seventeen million people:* Álvaro Moncayo and Antonio Carlos Silveira, "Current Epidemiological Trends for Chagas Disease in Latin America and Future Challenges in Epidemiology,

Surveillance and Health Policy," *Memórias do Instituto Oswaldo Cruz* 104, suppl. 1 (July 2009): 17–30.

PAGE 47 *She had kept a doll and a medal:* Kropf and Sá, "The Discovery of *Trypanosoma cruzi,*" 13–34; and João Amílcar Salgado, "The Centennial of Carlos Chagas and the Girl Berenice," *Memórias do Instituto Oswaldo Cruz,* 75 (1980): 193–195

PELEAS

PAGE 56 *The damage* T. cruzi *inflicts on the esophagus:* Fritz Köberle, "Chagas' Disease and Chagas' Syndromes: The Pathology of American Trypanosomiasis," *Advances in Parasitology* 6 (1968): 63–116.

IT SOUNDS WORSE IN SPANISH

PAGE 63 *That negative test results can be a mistake:* Diagnosing someone in the chronic stage of the kissing bug disease can be difficult in part because of the sensitivity of the tests and also perhaps because the parasite has distinct genetic lineages. Caryn Bern et al., "*Trypanosoma cruzi* and Chagas' Disease in the United States," *Clinical Microbiology Reviews* 24, no. 4 (October 2011): 670.

CALL IT GRIEF

PAGE 68 *I learned that the baby insects are called nymphs:* Herman Lent and Pedro W. Wygodzinsky, "Revision of the Triatominae (Hemiptera, Reduviidae), and Their Significance as Vectors of Chagas' Disease," *Bulletin of the American Museum of Natural History* 163, art. 3 (1979).

PAGE 69 *Although there are 140 species of these insects:* S. S. Catalá, F. Noireau, and J.-P. Dujardin, "Biology of Triatominae," in *American Trypanosomiasis, Chagas Disease: One Hundred Years of Research,* 2nd ed., eds. Jenny Telleria and Michel Tibayrenc (New York: Elsevier, 2017), p.145–46.

PAGE 69 *The faster a kissing bug defecates after biting:* Carolina E. Reisenman et al., "Feeding and Defecation Behavior of *Triatoma rubida* (Uhler, 1894) (Hemiptera: Reduviidae) under Laboratory Conditions, and Its Potential Role as a Vector of Chagas Disease in Arizona, USA," *American Journal of Tropical Medicine and Hygiene* 85, no. 4 (October 2011): 648–56.

PAGE 70 *Now I was reading that one study put the global cost:* Bruce Y. Lee et al., "Global Economic Burden of Chagas Disease: A Computational Simulation Model," *Lancet Infectious Diseases* 13, no. 4 (April 2013): 342–48.

PAGE 70 *If Tía Dora had arrived in the United States today:* Michael K. Gusmano, "Undocumented Immigrants in the United States: U.S. Health Policy and Access to Care," The Hastings Center, March 15, 2012.

PAGE 72 *Before the Affordable Care Act passed in 2010:* "Health Coverage by Race and Ethnicity: The Potential Impact of the Affordable Care Act," Henry J. Kaiser Family Foundation, March 13, 2013.

PAGE 72 *Now these women and men were waking up in European and American and Asian cities:* José Rodrigues Coura and Pedro Albajar Viñas, "Chagas Disease: A New Worldwide Challenge," *Nature* 465, no. 7301 (June 2010): S6–7.

INSECTARIO

PAGE 78 *Over the decades, he had, along with colleagues:* Felipe Guhl, Germán Aguilera, Néstor Pinto, and Daniela Vergara, "Actualización de la distribución geográfica y ecoepidemiología de la fauna de triatominos (Reduviidae: Triatominae) en Colombia," *Biomédica* 27, suppl. 1 (January 2007): 143–62.

page 78 *He had found that houses in close proximity:* Felipe Guhl, Nestor Pinto, and Germán Aguilera, "Sylvatic Triatominae: A New Challenge in Vector Control Transmission," *Memórias do Instituto Oswaldo Cruz* 104, suppl. 1 (July 2009): 71–75.

PAGE 79 *When Andean countries teamed in the nineties:* Felipe Guhl and Gustavo A. Vallejo, "Interruption of Chagas Disease Transmission in the Andean Countries: Colombia," *Memórias do Instituto Oswaldo Cruz* 94, suppl. 1 (September 1999): 413–15.

PAGE 79 *The study focused on the drug's effect on people:* Carlos A. Morillo et al., "Randomized Trial of Benznidazole for Chronic Chagas' Cardiomyopathy," *New England Journal of Medicine* 373, no. 14 (October 2015): 1295–306.

PAGE 79 *More than 60 percent of emerging infectious diseases:* Kate E. Jones, et al., "Global Trends in Emerging Infectious Diseases," *Nature*, 451 (February 2008): 990–994.

PAGE 80 *There are actually six genetic groups:* Simone Frédérique Brenière, Etienne Waleckx, and Christian Barnabé, "Over Six Thousand *Trypanosoma cruzi* Strains Classified into Discrete Typing Units (DTUs): Attempt at an Inventory," *PLOS Neglected Tropical Diseases* 10, no. 8 (August 2016).

PAGE 81 *Atacama is where astronomers go:* Simon Romero, "At the End of the Earth, Seeking Clues to the Universe," *New York Times*, April 7, 2012.

PAGE 81 *It's where scientists traveled with a telescope:* Dennis Overbye, "Darkness Visible, Finally: Astronomers Capture First Ever Image of a Black Hole," *New York Times*, April 10, 2019.

PAGE 81 *Atacama is also the place where military men:* Steven S. Volk, "Chile and the Traps of Memory," NACLA, June 30, 2011.

PAGE 81 *At Atacama, Professor Guhl and an international team:* Arthur C. Aufderheide et al., "A 9,000-year Record of Chagas' Disease," *Proceedings of the National Academy of Sciences* 101, no. 7 (February 2004): 2034–39.

PAGE 83 *I knew from reading articles that kissing bugs like the tempera-ture:* S. S. Catalá, F. Noireau, and J.-P. Dujardin, "Biology of Triatomi-nae," *in American Trypanosomiasis, Chagas Disease: One Hundred Years of Research*, 2nd ed., ed. Jenny Telleria and Michel Tibayrenc (New York: Elsevier, 2017), 149.

PAGE 83 *The first pair, located on the sides of the head:* Romina B. Bar-rozo et al., "An Inside Look at the Sensory Biology of Triatomines," *Journal of Insect Physiology* 97 (February 2017): 3–19.

PAGE 84 *nymphs, too, can transmit the parasite for the kissing bug disease:* Catalá, Noireau, and Dujardin, "Biology of Triatominae," 147

PAGE 84 *Bedbugs can harbor the parasite, and in the laboratory:* Renzo Salazar et al., "Bed Bugs (*Cimex lectularius*) as Vectors of *Trypanosoma cruzi*," *American Journal of Tropical Medicine and Hygiene* 92, no. 2 (February 2015): 331–35.

PAGE 85 *In 1995, when forty-two scientists and researchers from fifteen countries:* Felipe Guhl and C. J. Schofield, "Population Genetics and Con-trol of Triatominae," *Parasitology Today* 12, no. 5 (May 1996): 169–70.

PAGE 86 *According to the World Health Organization, the number of peo-ple infected:* For this and also information on government initiatives: J. C. P. Dias, A. C. Silveira, and C. J. Schofield, "The Impact of Chagas Disease Control in Latin America: A Review," *Memórias do Instituto Oswaldo Cruz* 97, no. 5 (July 2002): 603–12.

PAGE 86 children, *for reasons doctors do not fully understand, can often be cured:* Dr. Sergio Sosa-Estani (head of the Chagas Clinical Program, Drugs for Neglected Diseases Initiative) in discussion with the author, November 26, 2017; and Ana Lucia de Andrade, "Randomised Trial of Efficacy of Benznidazole in Treatment of Early *Trypanosoma cruzi* infec-tion," *Lancet* 348, Issue 9039: 1407–1413.

PAGE 86 *Maybe Latin America was winning the war against the disease:* Michael Barrett, "How the World Is Winning the Fight against Neglected Tropical Diseases," *New Statesman,* August 27, 2019.

PAGE 87 *Phil Gingrey, a congressman from Georgia, wrote to the CDC:* Cristina Marcos, "Gingrey: Child Migrants Pose Health Risk," *The Hill,* July 8, 2014.

PAGE 87 *He told an NBC reporter that Border Patrol agents:* *The Rachel Maddow Show,* transcript, MSNBC, aired July 15, 2014.

PAGE 87 *Americans turned away buses filled with migrant children:* Matt Hansen and Mark Boster, "Protesters in Murrieta Block Detainees' Buses in Tense Standoff," *Los Angeles Times,* July 1, 2014.

PAGE 87 *One picture taken by a Fox News photographer:* Tony Buttitta (@tonybuttitta), "Protesters appear to have stopped all buses trying to drop undocumented immigrants off in #Murietta. @myfoxla," Twitter photo, July 1, 2014.

PAGE 87 *The historian Alan M. Kraut calls it "medicalized nativism":* Alan M. Kraut, *Silent Travelers: Germs, Genes, and the "Immigrant Menace"* (New York: Basic Books, 1994), 2–3.

AUSTIN STATE HOSPITAL

I first learned of the racist medical experiment described in this chapter from parasitologist Robert S. Desowitz's *Who Gave Pinta to the Santa Maria? Torrid Diseases in a Temperate World* (New York: W. W. Norton & Company, 1997). Ardzroony Packchanian's correspondence, which I reviewed, can be found in his archives at the Truman G. Blocker, Jr. History of Medicine Collections in the Moody Medical Library at the University of Texas Medical Branch in Galveston. Details of the experiment depicted in this chapter come from A. Packchanian, "Infectivity of the Texas Strain of *Trypanosoma cruzi* to Man," *American Journal of Tropical Medicine and Hygienes* 1–23, no. 3 (May 1943): 309–14.

PAGE 90 *Since the institution's opening in 1861:* This and other details about the hospital are drawn from two sources: Sarah C. Sitton, *Life at the Texas State Lunatic Asylum, 1857–1997* (College Station, TX: Texas A&M University Press, 1999); and Ivan Belknap, *Human Problems of a State Mental Hospital* (New York: McGraw-Hill Book Company, 1956).

PAGE 91 *In Alabama, the Tuskegee syphilis study was underway:* DeNeen L. Brown, "'You've Got Bad Blood': The Horror of the Tuskegee Syphilis Experiment," *Washington Post,* May 16, 2017.

PAGE 91 *At Austin State Hospital, the young Black man was taken:* Packchanian's biographical sketch indicates that between 1936 and 1941 he was a protozoologist for the US Public Health Service. The sketch is published online by the Truman G. Blocker, Jr. History of Medicine Collections housed at the Moody Medical Library at the University of Texas Medical Branch in Galveston.

PAGE 91 *The researcher, Ardzroony Packchanian, had been asked to come to Texas:* Packchanian's obituary in the *Galveston Daily News,* May 8, 1987, states that "he was invited to study a few suspected cases of Chagas' disease." Correspondece shows that in one instance the Texas State Health Department turned over more than one thousand serum samples to him. Ardzroony Packchanian to Dr. J.V. Irons, 9 September 1948, box 6, folder 60, Truman G. Blocker, Jr. History of Medicine Collections, Moody Medical Library, University of Texas Medical Branch in Galveston.

PAGE 92 *A few years later, Congress passed annual quotas:* Mae M. Ngai, "The Architecture of Race in American Immigration Law: A Reexamination of the Immigration Act of 1924," *Journal of American History* 86, no. 1 (June 1999): 74.

PAGE 92 *He enrolled at the City College of New York:* "Dr. A.A. Packchanian," *Galveston Daily News,* May 8, 1987.

PAGE 92 *He completed his doctoral work on sleeping sickness:* Ardzroony Packchanian, "Experimental *Trypanosoma brucei* Infection and Immunity in Various Species of Animals; Blood Chemistry and Electrical Conductivity of Nagana Blood" (PhD diss., University of Michigan, 1933).

PAGE 92 *News of his research had appeared in the* New York Times: "'Kissing Bug' Accused," *New York Times*, August 26, 1939.

PAGE 95 *In the 1940s, though, such antibody tests did not exist:* A. O. Luquetti and G. A. Schmuñis, "Diagnosis of *Trypanosoma cruzi* Infection," in *American Trypanosomiasis, Chagas Disease: One Hundred Years of Research*, 2nd ed., eds. Jenny Telleria and Michel Tibayrenc (New York: Elsevier, 2017), 679.

PAGE 95 *And he spent a decade looking for people:* Ardzroony Packchanian to Piero Manginelli, April 2, 1951, box 6, folder 61, Truman G. Blocker, Jr. History of Medicine Collection, Moody Medical Library, University of Texas Medical Branch in Galveston.

PAGE 95 *He wanted to know what had come of Packchanian's experiments:* Garland G. Zedler to Ardzroony Packchanian, March 5, 1946, box 6, folder 60, Truman G. Blocker, Jr. History of Medicine Collection, Moody Medical Library, University of Texas Medical Branch in Galveston.

PHARMA BRO

PAGE 97 *My sister had moved to Virginia where the Latinx population:* Carole Morello and Dan Keating. "Va.'s Numbers of Hispanics and Asians Skyrocket as White Population Dwindles," *Washington Post*, February 4, 2011.

PAGE 97 *Donald Trump, then the leading Republican presidential candidate:* Bethany McLean, "Poison Pill," *Vanity Fair*, February 2016.

PAGE 97 *In the fall of 2015, Shkreli's company hiked the price:* Andrew Pollack, "Drug Goes from $13.50 a Tablet to $750, Overnight," *New York Times,* September 20, 2015.

PAGE 98 *Immigrants, black Americans, and those living in poverty are more likely:* Jeffrey L. Jones et al., *"Toxoplasma gondii* Infection in the United States, 2011–2014," *American Journal of Tropical Medicine and Hygiene* 98, no. 2 (February 2018): 551–57.

PAGE 98 *He went on Bloomberg Television and defended the price increase:* Jared S. Hopkins, "Controversial 'Pharma Bro' Shkreli Says 'Of Course' He'd Raise Drug Price Again," *Bloomberg,* December 23, 2016.

PAGE 98 *He showed up at the Forbes Healthcare Summit:* Dan Diamond, "Martin Shkreli Admits He Messed Up: He Should've Raised Prices Even Higher," *Forbes,* December 3, 2015.

PAGE 98 *He then spent $2 million on the only existing copy of a Wu-Tang Clan album:* Justin Hunte, "Martin Shkreli Plans to Bail-Out Bobby Shmurda," HipHopDx.com, December 16, 2015.

PAGE 98 *That same year, executives from Valeant Pharmaceuticals:* Pollack, "Drug Goes from $13.50 a Tablet," *New York Times.*

PAGE 98 *A year later, the pharmaceutical company Mylan:* Andrew Pollack, "Mylan Raised EpiPen's Price Before the Expected Arrival of a Generic," *New York Times,* August 24, 2016.

PAGE 99 *a man who, in the summer of 2015, at the age of thirty-two, could:* Diana Novak Jones, "Shkreli's Ex-Co. OK to Pay $198K in Bonuses, Judge Says," Law360, February 17, 2016.

PAGE 99 *The World Health Organization considers benznidazole:* World Health Organization Model List of Essential Medicines, 21st list (Geneva: World Health Organization, 2019).

NOTES

PAGE 99 *The drug can often eradicate the parasite:* Maria Carmo Pereira Nunes et al., "Chagas Cardiomyopathy: An Update of Current Clinical Knowledge and Management: A Scientific Statement from the American Heart Association," *Circulation* 138, no. 12 (September 2018): e169–e209.

PAGE 99 *Studies have also found that women treated with benznidazole:* Diana L. Fabbro et al., "Trypanocide Treatment of Women Infected with *Trypanosoma cruzi* and Its Effect on Preventing Congenital Chagas," *PLOS Neglected Tropical Diseases* 8, no. 11 (November 20, 2014): e3312; and Sergio Sosa-Estani et al., "Etiological Treatment of Young Women Infected with *Trypanosoma cruzi*, and Prevention of Congenital Transmission," *Revista da Sociedade Brasileira de Medicina Tropical* 42, no. 5 (September/October 2009): 484–87.

PAGE 100 *Benznidazole, which interferes with the parasite's protein synthesis:* Constança Britto (director, Molecular Biology and Endemic Diseases Laboratory, Oswaldo Cruz Institute) in discussion with the author, November 13, 2019.

PAGE 100 *this might explain why an observational study in Argentina:* Rodolfo Viotti et al., "Long-Term Cardiac Outcomes of Treating Chronic Chagas Disease with Benznidazole Versus No Treatment: A Nonrandomized Trial," *Annals of Internal Medicine* 144, no. 10 (May 2006): 724–34.

PAGE 100 *The study that Professor Guhl had been working on:* Carlos A. Morillo et al., "Randomized Trial of Benznidazole for Chronic Chagas' Cardiomyopathy," *New England Journal of Medicine* 373, no. 14 (October 2015): 1295–1306.

PAGE 100 *In 2015, benznidazole was not approved by the US Food and Drug Administration:* Caryn Bern, "Chagas' Disease," *New England Journal of Medicine* 373, no. 5 (July 2015): 456–66.

NOTES

PAGE 100 *Martin Shkreli bragged to investors that his company:* This and other details about Shkreli's plans and proposed price hike are from my reporting for "Pharma Bro's Latest Move Targets Latinos," *Atlantic*, December 14, 2015; and Pollack, "Martin Shkreli's Latest Plan to Sharply Raise Drug Price Prompts Outcry," *New York Times.*

PAGE 100 *He boasted that this would generate millions of dollars:* Helen Branswell, "How a System Meant to Develop Drugs for Rare Diseases Broke Down," STAT, November 28, 2015.

PAGE 100 *One study led by a clinical fellow from Harvard Medical School:* Jennifer Manne-Goehler, Michael R. Reich, and Veronika J. Wirtz, "Access to Care for Chagas Disease in the United States: A Health Systems Analysis," *American Journal of Tropical Medicine and Hygiene* 93, no. 1 (May 2015): 108–13.

PAGE 101 *In South America, the cost of treatment with benznidazole:* Andrew Pollack, "Martin Shkreli's Latest Plan to Sharply Raise Drug Price Prompts Outcry," *New York Times*, December 11, 2015.

PAGE 101 *It also didn't charge for another drug, nifurtimox:* Jennifer Manne et al., "Supply Chain Problems for Chagas Disease Treatment," *Lancet Infectious Diseases* 12, no. 3 (March 2012): 173–75.

PAGE 101 *This drug was often not as well tolerated as benznidazole:* Nunes et al., "Chagas Cardiomyopathy: An Update."

PAGE 101 *Investors gave his company $8 million in the hopes:* Jones, "Shkreli's Ex-Co. OK to Pay."

PAGE 101 *The morning after Shkreli and I exchanged tweets:* Christie Smythe and Keri Geiger, "Shkreli, Drug Price Gouger, Denies Fraud and Posts Bail," *Bloomberg News*, December 17, 2015.

PAGE 103 Harper's *documented how Shkreli's notoriety:* "Public Enemy," *Harper's*, September 2017.

PAGE 103 *It got a new president and later a new name:* Ron Leuty, "Pharma Bad Boy Martin Shkreli Is Gone, But 2 Companies Spark Over Drug He Snagged," *San Francisco Business Times*, August 4, 2017.

HUNTING FOR THE KISSING BUG

PAGE 107 *In 2013, she and her team screened more than two hundred shelter dogs:* Trevor D. Tenney et al., "Shelter Dogs as Sentinels for *Trypanosoma cruzi* Transmission across Texas," *Emerging Infectious Diseases* 20, no. 8 (August 2014): 1323–26.

PAGE 107 *When—and if—the symptoms of the kissing bug disease show themselves:* Dr. Roy Madigan (Animal Hospital of Smithson Valley) in discussion with the author, December 20, 2018.

PAGE 108 *In the late 1970s, the state's health department and Pan American University:* J. E. Burkholder, T. C. Allison, and V. P. Kelly, "*Trypanosoma cruzi* (Chagas) (Protozoa: Kinetoplastida) in Invertebrate, Reservoir, and Human Hosts of the Lower Rio Grande Valley of Texas," *Journal of Parasitology* 66, no. 2 (April 1980): 305–11.

PAGE 108 *Almost thirty years later, in 2008, Sonia Kjos:* S. A. Kjos et al., "Distribution and Characterization of Canine Chagas Disease in Texas," *Veterinary Parasitology* 152, no. 3–4 (April 2008): 249–56.

PAGE 108 *Infected dogs have also been found in Oklahoma, Louisiana, and Virginia:* P. D. Nieto et al., "Comparison of Two Immunochromatographic Assays and the Indirect Immunofluorescence Antibody Test for Diagnosis of *Trypanosoma cruzi* Infection in Dogs in South Central Louisiana," *Veterinary Parasitology* 165, no. 3–4 (November 2009): 241–47; Kristy K. Bradley et al., "Prevalence of American Trypanosomiasis (Chagas Disease) among Dogs in Oklahoma," *Journal of the American Veterinary Medical Association* 217, no. 12 (December 2000): 1853–57; and S. C. Barr et al., "*Trypanosoma cruzi* Infection in Walker Hounds from Virginia," *American Journal of Veterinary Research* 56, no. 8 (August 1995): 1037–44.

PAGE 108 *In 2015, Melissa Nolan Garcia, an epidemiologist at Baylor College:* Melissa N. Garcia et al., "Case Report: Evidence of Autochthonous Chagas Disease in Southeastern Texas," *American Journal of Tropical Medicine and Hygiene* 92, no. 2 (February 2015): 325–30.

PAGE 109 *When I started digging through medical journals:* Kathryn M. Meurs et al., "Chronic *Trypanosoma cruzi* Infection in Dogs: 11 Cases (1987–1996)," *Journal of the American Veterinary Medical Association* 213, no. 4 (August 1998): 497–500.

PAGE 111 *In 2003, researchers found DNA evidence:* Karl Reinhard, T. Michael Fink, and Jack Skiles, "A Case of Megacolon in Rio Grande Valley as a Possible Case of Chagas Disease," *Memórias do Instituto Oswaldo Cruz* 98, suppl. 1 (January 2003): 165–72; and Adauto Araújo et al., "Paleoparasitology of Chagas Disease: A Review," *Memórias do Instituto Oswaldo Cruz* 104, suppl. 1 (July 2009): 9–16.

PAGE 112 *By 2016, they had a collection of almost two thousand bugs:* Rachel Curtis-Robles et al., "Combining Public Health Education and Disease Ecology Research: Using Citizen Science to Assess Chagas Disease Entomological Risk in Texas," *PLOS Neglected Tropical Diseases* 9, no. 12 (December 2015).

THE MILITARY'S SEARCH

PAGE 117 *The United States military began hunting for kissing bugs in 1964:* Warren Floyd Pippin, "The Biology and Vector Capability of *Triatoma sanguisuga texana* Usinger and *Triatoma gerstaeckeri* (Stål) Compared with *Rhodnius prolixus* (Stål) (Hemiptera: Triatominae)," *Journal of Medical Entomology* 7, no. 1 (January 1970): 30–45.

PAGE 118 *In 2012, the US military published a study:* Lee McPhatter et al., "Vector Surveillance to Determine Species Composition and Occurrence of *Trypanosoma cruzi* Infection at Three Military Installations in San Antonio, Texas," *US Army Medical Department Journal* (July–September 2012): 12–21.

PAGE 118 *When Dr. Hamer and her team tested almost two thousand kissing bugs:* Rachel Curtis-Robles et al., "Combining Public Health Education and Disease Ecology Research: Using Citizen Science to Assess Chagas Disease Entomological Risk in Texas," *PLOS Neglected Tropical Diseases* 9, no. 12 (December 2015).

PAGE 118 *In 2018, it also had the highest rate of poverty:* Camille Phillips, "San Antonio Poverty Rate Tops List of Large Metro Areas," Texas Public Radio, September 26, 2019.

PAGE 118 *close to 14 percent of the dogs in the city's shelters:* Trevor D. Tenney et al., "Shelter Dogs as Sentinels for *Trypanosoma cruzi* Transmission across Texas," *Emerging Infectious Diseases* 20, no. 8 (August 2014): 1323–26.

PAGE 119 *"A fully trained military dog costs":* Kyle Stock, "The Dogs of War Are in High Demand," *Bloomberg,* August 28, 2017.

PAGE 119 *In 2016, the military had approximately 1,800 dogs: Department of Defense: Medical Conditions and Care for End of-Service Military Working Dogs* (Washington, DC: United States Government Accountability Office, 2017).

PAGE 119 *A retired dog handler told the* San Antonio Express-News: Cathy M. Rosenthal, "Animals Matter: Military Working Dogs Still Considered 'Equipment,'" *San Antonio Express-News,* April 3, 2013.

PAGE 119 *In the late seventies, a Labrador retriever at Lackland:* John M. Pletcher and Harold W. Casey, "Case for Diagnosis," *Military Medicine* 143, no. 10 (October 1978): 689–94.

PAGE 120 *Veterinarians at Lackland began reporting more cases:* McPhatter et al., "Vector Surveillance to Determine Species Composition," 12–21. This source also includes more information about the infection rates among these dogs.

PAGE 121 *Between 2014 and 2016, the military screened:* Joseph E. Marcus et al., "Diagnostic Evaluation of Military Blood Donors Screening Positive for *Trypanosoma cruzi* Infection," *Medical Surveillance Monthly Report* 25, no. 2 (February 2018): 16–19.

PAGE 121 *They included an eighteen-year-old who already:* Bryant J. Webber et al., "A Case of Chagas Cardiomyopathy Following Infection in South Central Texas," *United States Army Medical Department Journal* (January–June 2017): 55–59.

PAGE 121 *After living in the exact location for thirteen years:* Sonia A. Kjos et al., "Identification of Bloodmeal Sources and *Trypanosoma cruzi* Infection in Triatomine Bugs (Hemiptera: Reduviidae) from Residential Settings in Texas, the United States," *Journal of Medical Entomology* 50, no. 5 (September 2013): 1126–39.

PAGE 122 *The family noticed this uptick around the same time:* McPhatter et al., "Vector Surveillance to Determine Species Composition," 12–21.

PAGE 122 *Starting in the late nineties, Texas had more than a million acres:* Texas A&M Institute of Renewable Natural Resources, "Status Update and Trends of Texas Rural Working Lands," *Texas Land Trends* 1, no. 1 (October 2014): 2.

PAGE 122 *between 2010 and 2017, it had added more housing than any other state:* US Census Bureau, "Census Bureau Reveals Fastest-Growing Large Cities," release no. CB18-78, May 24, 2018.

PAGE 122 *In 2018, Apple announced it was building:* Will Anderson, "A Primer on Robinson Ranch, 7,000 Acres of Central Texas That Will Be Home to New $1B Apple Campus," *Austin Business Journal*, December 15, 2018.

PAGE 122 *Insects that carry disease are usually sensitive to temperature shifts:* A. Marm Kilpatrick and Sarah E. Randolph, "Drivers, Dynamics, and Control of Emerging Vector-Borne Zoonotic Diseases," *Lancet* 380, no. 9857 (December 2012): 1946–1955.

PAGE 122 *kissing bugs tend to feed more frequently:* S. S. Catalá, F. Noireau, and J.-P. Dujardin, "Biology of Triatominae," in *American Trypanosomiasis, Chagas Disease: One Hundred Years of Research,* 2nd ed., eds. Jenny Telleria and Michel Tibayrenc (New York: Elsevier, 2017), 149.

PAGE 122 *That said, scientists have pointed out that it is hard to isolate:* Kilpatrick and Randolph, "Drivers, Dynamics, and Control of Emerging Vector-Borne Zoonotic Diseases," 1946–55.

PAGE 123 *In Chile, one group of researchers mapped the risk:* Salvador Ayala et al., "Estimando el efecto del cambio climático sobre el riesgo de la enfermedad de Chagas en Chile por medio del número reproductivo," *Revista Médica de Chile* 147, no. 6 (June 2019): 683–692.

PAGE 123 *Argentinian researchers looked at five species:* Soledad Ceccarelli and Jorge E. Rabinovich, "Global Climate Change Effects on Venezuela's Vulnerability to Chagas Disease is Linked to the Geographic Distribution of Five Triatomine Species," *Journal of Medical Entomology* 52, no. 6 (November 2015): 1333–43.

PAGE 123 *In 2013, researchers from the University of Texas-Pan American:* Miroslava Garza et al., "Projected Future Distributions of Vectors of *Trypanosoma cruzi* in North America under Climate Change Scenarios," *PLOS Neglected Tropical Diseases* 8, no. 5 (2014): e2818.

PAGE 123 *In 2015, the CDC granted Texas researchers:* "Texas Medical Center, UTHealth Researcher Awarded CDC Grant to Study Chagas Disease in Texas," press release, September 14, 2015.

PAGE 123 *It was part of an initiative to tackle a handful:* Centers for Disease Control and Prevention, "Parasitic Infections Also Occur in the United States," press release, May 8, 2014.

PAGE 124 *The list of neglected parasitic infections includes:* Jeffrey L. Jones et al., "*Toxoplasma gondii* Infection in the United States, 2011–2014," *American Journal of Tropical Medicine and Hygiene* 98, no. 2 (February 2018): 551–57.

PAGE 124 *Also on the list: toxocariasis, a disease caused by:* Kathleen McAuliffe, *This Is Your Brain on Parasites: How Tiny Creatures Manipulate Our Behavior and Shape Society* (New York: Houghton Mifflin Harcourt, 2016), 94; and A. Farmer, T. Beltran, and Y. S. Choi, "Prevalence of Toxocara Species Infection in the U.S.: Results from the National Health and Nutrition Examination Survey, 2011–2014," *PLOS Neglected Tropical Diseases* 11, no. 7 (July 2017).

PAGE 124 *Every year, the disease blinds at least seventy people:* Centers for Disease Control and Prevention, "Parasitic Infections Also Occur in the United States," 2014.

PAGE 125 *A year after the grants were announced, a study:* Jennifer Manne-Goehler et al., "Estimating the Burden of Chagas Disease in the United States," *PLOS Neglected Tropical Diseases* 10, no. 11 (November 2016).

PAGE 125 *The CDC has recorded fewer than a hundred such infections:* Centers for Disease Control and Prevention, email message to author, April 20, 2020.

PAGE 126 *She had more than fifty bites from kissing bugs:* Patricia L. Dorn et al., "Autochthonous Transmission of *Trypanosoma cruzi*, Louisiana," *Emerging Infectious Diseases* 13, no. 4 (April 2007): 605–7.

PAGE 126 *Researchers screened more than a hundred women and men:* Nicole Behrens-Bradley et al., "Kissing Bugs Harboring *Trypanosoma cruzi*, Frequently Bite Residents of the US Southwest But Do Not Cause Chagas Disease," *American Journal of Medicine* 133, no. 1 (January 2020): 108–114.

IF TÍA HAD KNOWN

For a lively introduction to parasites, see Carl Zimmer, *Parasite Rex: Inside the Bizarre World of Nature's Most Dangerous Creatures* (New York: Atria, 2000).

PAGE 129 *In the belly of a kissing bug, it looks like a tadpole with a pointed face:* "Parasites - American Trypanosomiasis (also known as Chagas Disease)," Centers for Disease Control and Prevention, updated February 11, 2019, https://www.cdc.gov/parasites/chagas/; W. de Souza, T. U. de Carvalho, and E. S. Barrias, "Ultrastructure of *Trypanosoma cruzi* and Its Interaction with Host Cells," in *American Trypanosomiasis, Chagas Disease: One Hundred Years of Research*, 2nd ed., eds. Jenny Telleria and Michel Tibayrenc (New York: Elsevier, 2017), 401–28; and Wanderley de Souza, "Electron Microscopy of Trypanosomes: A Historical View," *Memórias do Instituto Oswaldo Cruz* 103, no. 4 (June 2008): 313–25.

PAGE 129 *From the Greek,* trypanon *means a borer:* Centers for Disease Control and Prevention, "Etymologia: *Trypanosoma*," *Emerging Infectious Diseases* 12, no. 9 (September 2006): 1473.

PAGE 131 *After much testing, Dr. Kirchhoff and Otsu figured out:* Louis Kirchhoff and Keiko Otsu. Recombinant Polypeptides for Diagnosing Infection with *Trypanosoma cruzi*. US Patent 7,491,515 B2, filed December 4, 2001, and issued February 17, 2009.

PAGE 131 *He licensed the proteins to Abbott Diagnostics:* "Trypanosoma cruzi (T. cruzi) (Anti-T. cruzi Assay)," US Food and Drug Administration, updated April 11, 2019, https://www.fda.gov/vaccines-blood-biologics/blood-donor-screening/trypanosoma-cruzi-t-cruzi-anti-t-cruzi-assay.

JANET AND HER BABY

Although the physician who oversaw the care for Janet's baby denied my requests for interviews, a case report about the newborn was published and this provided the medical information for this chapter: Andrés Alarcón et al., "Diagnosis and Treatment of Congenital Chagas Disease in a Premature Infant," *Journal of the Pediatric Infectious Diseases Society* 5, no. 4 (December 2016): e28–e31.

PAGE 143 *It's called congenital Chagas disease:* Morven S. Edwards et al., "Perinatal Screening for Chagas Disease in Southern Texas," *Journal of the Pediatric Infectious Diseases Society* 4, no. 1 (March 2015): 67–70.

PAGE 143 *Such a transmission happened in Washington, DC:* Louis V. Kirchhoff, Albert A. Gam, and Flora C. Gilliam, "American Trypanosomiasis (Chagas' Disease) in Central American Immigrants," *American Journal of Medicine* 82, no. 5 (May 1987): 915–20.

PAGE 144 *The CDC estimates that anywhere between 63 and 315 babies:* Susan P. Montgomery et al., "Neglected Parasitic Infections in the United States: Chagas Disease," *American Journal of Tropical Medicine and Hygiene* 90, no. 5 (May 2014): 814–18.

PAGE 144 *In Latin America, the numbers are much higher:* Pan American Health Organization/World Health Organization, "PAHO Launches New Initiative to Eliminate Mother-to-Child Transmission of Four Diseases," press release, August 10, 2017.

PAGE 144 *If they were, many of the lost babies could be saved:* Maria Carmo Pereira Nunes et al., "Chagas Cardiomyopathy: An Update of Current Clinical Knowledge and Management: A Scientific Statement from the American Heart Association," *Circulation* 138, no. 12 (September 2018): e191.

PAGE 144 *According to the Pan American Health Organization, about one-third:* Pan American Health Organization/World Health Organization, "PAHO Launches New Initiative to Eliminate Mother-to-Child Transmission of Four Diseases."

PAGE 144 *In 2013, a man in his early twenties showed up:* Jorge Murillo et al., "Congenital Chagas' Disease Transmission in the United States: Diagnosis in Adulthood," *ID Cases* 5 (2016): 72–75.

PAGE 144 *In 2010, the year Tía Dora died, a boy in Virginia:* Raul A. Lazarte et al., "Congenital Transmission of Chagas Disease—Virginia, 2010," *Morbidity and Mortality Weekly Report* 61, no. 26 (July 6, 2012): 477–79.

PAGE 154 *While the percentage of children born with congenital form:* Louisa Messenger and Caryn Bern, "Congenital Chagas Disease: Current Diagnostics, Limitations and Future Perspectives," *Current Opinion in Infectious Diseases* 31, no. 5 (October 2018): 415–421.

PAGE 154 *in one area of Janet's home country, a study estimated that about 7 percent:* Caryn Bern, Diana L. Martin, and Robert H. Gilman, "Acute and Congenital Chagas Disease," *Advances in Parasitology* 75, (2011): 30.

PAGE 158 *The correct answer is yes, but 84 percent of obstetricians and gynecologists:* Jennifer R. Verani et al., "Survey of Obstetrician-Gynecologists in the United States about Chagas Disease," *American Journal of Tropical Medicine and Hygiene* 83, no. 4 (October 2010): 891–95.

PAGE 158 *almost seven hundred thousand babies are born every year:* "Number of Births by Hispanic Origin of Mother," State Health Facts, Henry J. Kaiser Family Foundation, 2017.

PAGE 158 *In 2006, the federal government convened a panel of experts:* Michael Watson et al., "Newborn Screening: Toward a Uniform Screening Panel and System—Executive Summary," *Pediatrics* 117, suppl. 3 (May 2006): S296–S307.

PAGE 158 *Newborns are screened for fifteen diseases that occur less frequently:* R. Rodney Howell et al., "CDC Grand Rounds: Newborn Screening and Improved Outcomes," *Morbidity and Mortality Weekly Report* 61, no. 21 (June 1, 2012): 390–93; and Edwards et al., "Perinatal Screening for Chagas Disease in Southern Texas," *Journal of the Pediatric Infectious Diseases Society* 4, no. 1 (March 2015): 67–70.

PAGE 158 *Eileen Stillwaggon, an economist at Gettysburg College:* Eileen Stillwaggon et al., "Congenital Chagas Disease in the United States: Cost Savings through Maternal Screening," *American Journal of Tropical Medicine and Hygiene* 98, no. 6 (June 2018): 1733–42.

PAGE 158 *A girl infected with the kissing bug disease, like Janet:* Sergio Sosa-Estani et al., "Etiological Treatment of Young Women Infected with *Trypanosoma cruzi*, and Prevention of Congenital Transmission," *Revista da Sociedade Brasileira de Medicina Tropical* 42, no. 5 (September/October 2009): 484–87.

LA DOCTORA

PAGE 161 *The FDA had not approved benznidazole for use in the United States:* Andrés Alarcón et al., "Diagnosis and Treatment of Congenital Chagas Disease in a Premature Infant," *Journal of the Pediatric Infectious Diseases Society* 5, no. 4 (December 2016): e28–e31.

PAGE 162 *She would have started on medication:* I based this upon what I witnessed for patients whose stories I document elsewhere in this book. Also see: Caryn Bern, "Chagas' Disease," *New England Journal of Medicine* 373, no. 5 (July 2015): 456–66.

PAGE 166 *Adults can have allergic reactions:* US Food and Drug Administration, "Benznidazole Tablets, for Oral Use," August 2017.

CANDACE

PAGE 169 *She was one of at least seventy-five people:* Centers for Disease Control and Prevention, email message to author, April 20, 2020.

PAGE 173 *The sanitary engineer who traced the typhoid outbreak:* For this and other details about Mallon, see: Priscilla Wald, *Contagious: Cultures, Carriers, and the Outbreak Narrative* (Durham, North Carolina: Duke University Press, 2008), 84–107; and Alan M. Kraut, *Silent Travelers: Germs, Genes, and the "Immigrant Menace"* (New York: Basic Books, 1994), 98–103.

PAGE 174 *The CDC erroneously labeled Haitians a high-risk group:* Edwidge Danticat, "Trump Reopens an Old Wound for Haitians," *The New Yorker,* December 29, 2017.

PAGE 175 *A search in PubMed, the medical literature database, confirmed:* Norman C. Woody and Hannah B. Woody, "American Trypanosomiasis (Chagas' disease); First Indigenous Case in the United States," *Journal of the American Medical Association* 159, no. 7 (October 15, 1955): 676–77.

PAGE 177 *A year after the baby was diagnosed, a dermatology journal:* T. L. Shields and E. N. Walsh, "'Kissing Bug' Bite," *Archives of Dermatology* 74, no. 1 (July 1956): 14–21.

PAGE 177 *Seven children were infected:* Norman C. Woody, Noel De-Dianous, and Hannah B. Woody, "American Trypanosomiasis: II. Current Serologic Studies in Chagas' Disease," *Journal of Pediatrics* 58, no. 5 (May 1961): 738–45.

PAGE 177 *Researchers screened Native Americans:* P. T. K. Woo, "Mammalian Trypanosomiasis and Piscine Cryptobiosis in Canada and the United States," *Bulletin of the Society of Vector Ecology* 16, no. 1 (June 1991): 25–42.

PAGE 177 *In 1982, kissing bugs in Northern California bit a woman:* T. R. Navin et al., "Human and Sylvatic *Trypanosoma cruzi* Infection in California," *American Journal of Public Health* 75, no. 4 (April 1985): 366–69.

PAGE 177 *A year later, in 1983, a newborn in Corpus Christi:* Diane E. Ochs et al., "Postmortem Diagnosis of Autochthonous Acute Chagasic Myocarditis by Polymerase Chain Reaction Amplification of a Species-Specific DNA Sequence of *Trypanosoma cruzi,*" *American Journal of Tropical Medicine and Hygiene* 54, no. 5 (May 1996): 526–29.

PAGE 177 *The following year, Violette S. Hnilica, a pathologist:* Ochs et al., "Postmortem Diagnosis of Autochthonous Acute Chagasic Myocarditis," 526–29.

PAGE 178 *When Texas health officials arrived at the family's home:* Texas Department of Health, "Chagas' Disease Investigation," *Texas Preventable Disease* News 44, no. 31 (August 4, 1984).

MAIRA

PAGE 84 *Maira had an advantage over the parasite:* Elizabeth Whitman, "Chagas Disease: How a Silent Tropical Parasite Prospers in the US," *International Business Times,* May 26, 2015.

PAGE 184 *California has the highest number of people:* Jennifer Manne-Goehler et al., "Estimating the Burden of Chagas Disease in the United States," *PLOS Neglected Tropical Diseases* 10, no. 11 (November 2016).

PAGE 186 *She didn't know that every year an estimated ten thousand people die:* "Chagas Disease (American Trypanosomiasis)," World Health Organization, https://www.who.int/chagas/epidemiology/en/.

PAGE 186 *One study in Brazil looked at blood samples:* Ligia Capuani et al., "Mortality among Blood Donors Seropositive and Seronegative for Chagas Disease (1996–2000) in São Paulo, Brazil: A Death Certificate Linkage Study," *PLOS Neglected Tropical Diseases* 11, no. 5 (May 2017).

PAGE 187 *About 66 percent of the hospital's patients hailed from Latin America:* Anne Robinson (compliance and privacy officer, Olive View-UCLA Medical Center), email message to author, October 26, 2016.

PAGE 187 *two-thirds of the patients at Olive View did not have health insurance:* Esmeralda Bermudez and Alexandra Zavis, "Olive View Sees Healthcare Ruling as a New Challenge," *Los Angeles Times,* June 29, 2012.

PAGE 187 *A study published in 2018 looked closely at fifty of Dr. Meymandi's patients:* Colin Forsyth et al., "'It's Like a Phantom Disease': Patient Perspectives on Access to Treatment for Chagas Disease in the United States," *American Journal of Tropical Medicine and Hygiene* 98, no 3 (March 2018): 735–41.

PAGE 189 *raping the children, selling them to illegal adoption networks:* Associated Press, "Soldiers Stole Children During El Salvador's war," February 22, 2013; and Larry Rohter. "El Salvador's Stolen Children Face a War's Darkest Secret," *New York Times,* August 5, 1996.

PAGE 189 *That's when the letter from a blood donation center arrived:* Maira was most likely part of a study led by the American Red Cross to assess the risk of *T. cruzi* among Latin American immigrant blood donors. David A. Leiby et al., "*Trypanosoma cruzi* in Los Angeles and Miami Blood Donors: Impact of Evolving Donor Demographics on Seroprevalence and Implications for Transfusion Transmission," *Transfusion* 42, no. 5 (June 2002): 549–55.

PAGE 192 *The few times major media outlets:* Andrew Pollack, "Martin Shkreli's Latest Plan to Sharply Raise Drug Price Prompts Outcry," *New York Times,* December 11, 2015; and "'Neglected Infections' Resurface Among America's Poor," *PBS NewsHour,* transcript, PBS, aired October 27, 2009.

PAGE 192 *Dr. Meymandi found that close to 14 percent:* Sheba K. Meymandi et al., "Prevalence of Chagas Disease in Los Angeles Latin American Immigrant Population with Cardiomyopathy," *Journal of Cardiac Failure* 14, no. 6S, suppl. (August 2008): S1–S128.

PAGE 192 *A 2013 study in two New York City hospitals found similar results:* Luciano Kapelusznik et al., "Chagas Disease in Latin American Immigrants with Dilated Cardiomyopathy in New York City," *Clinical Infectious Diseases* 57, no. 1 (July 2013): e7.

PAGE 193 *Dr. Meymandi and her colleagues tested close to five thousand people:* Sheba K. Meymandi et al., "Prevalence of Chagas Disease in the Latin American-Born Population of Los Angeles," *Clinical Infectious Diseases* 64, no. 9 (May 2017): 1182–88.

PAGE 195 *about 7 percent of the Latin American patients with pacemakers:* Sandy Park et al., "The Prevalence of Chagas Disease among Latin American Immigrants with Pacemakers in Los Angeles, California," *American Journal of Tropical Medicine and Hygiene* 96, no. 5 (May 2017): 1139–42.

PAGE 196 *Consider lymphatic filariasis, a disease caused by worms:* "Lymphatic Filariasis," World Health Organization, https://www.who.int/news-room/fact-sheets/detail/lymphatic-filariasis.

PAGE 196 *The rate of people with the kissing bug disease had been on the decline:* Kevin M. Bonney, "Chagas Disease in the 21st Century: A Public Health Success or an Emerging Threat?" *Parasite* 21, no. 11 (March 2014).

PAGE 196 *The same was true of lymphatic filariasis:* World Health Organization, "Global Programme to Eliminate Lymphatic Filariasis: Progress Report, 2016," *Weekly Epidemiological Record* 92, no. 40 (October 2017): 594–608.

CARLOS

PAGE 207 *One team of CDC experts and infectious disease specialists:* Elizabeth B. Gray et al., "Reactivation of Chagas Disease among Heart Transplant Recipients in the United States, 2012–2016," *Transplant Infectious Disease* 20, no. 6 (December 2018): e12996.

PAGE 208 *There's speculation that the drugs used to keep the body:* Reinaldo B. Bestetti and Tatiana Theodoropoulos, "A Systematic Review of Studies on Heart Transplantation for Patients with End-Stage Chagas' Heart Disease," *Journal of Cardiac Failure* 15, no. 3 (April 2009): 249–55.

NOTES

CHURCH BASEMENT

PAGE 215 *Back in the 1980s, he had screened 205 people:* Louis V. Kirchhoff, Albert A. Gam, and Flora C. Gilliam, "American Trypanosomiasis (Chagas' Disease) in Central American Immigrants," *American Journal of Medicine* 82, no. 5 (May 1987): 915–20.

PAGE 216 *Blood banks do not check repeat donors:* US Food and Drug Administration, *Use of Serological Tests to Reduce the Risk of Transmission of* Trypanosoma cruzi *Infection in Blood and Blood Components* (Silver Spring, MD: Office of Communication, Outreach and Development, 2017).

PAGE 216 *The CDC considers a person to have the disease:* Centers for Disease Control and Prevention, "DPDx - Laboratory Identification of Parasites of Public Health Concern," updated April 30, 2019.

PAGE 217 *The FDA would approve the first rapid test:* Jeffrey D. Whitman et al., "Chagas Disease Serological Test Performance in U.S. Blood Donor Specimens," *Journal of Clinical Microbiology* 57, no. 12 (November 2019).

PAGE 217 *A few studies in Latin America produced mixed results:* Claudia L. Sánchez-Camargo et al., "Comparative Evaluation of 11 Commercialized Rapid Diagnostic Tests for Detecting *Trypanosoma cruzi* Antibodies in Serum Banks in Areas of Endemicity and Nonendemicity," *Journal of Clinical Microbiology* 52, no. 7 (July 2014): 2506–12; and Karina E. Egüez et al., "Rapid Diagnostic Tests Duo as Alternative to Conventional Serological Assays for Conclusive Chagas Disease Diagnosis," *PLOS Neglected Tropical Diseases* 11, no. 4 (April 3, 2017).

PAGE 220 *Where he worked was a region of South America:* Peter Hotez, "Chagas Disease: The New Numbers," *Speaking of Medicine* (blog), *PLOS*, March 3, 2015.

THE GREAT EPI DIVIDE

PAGE 225 *In the eighties and nineties, thanks to activists:* Nurith Aizenman, "How to Demand a Medical Breakthrough: Lessons from the AIDS Fight," WBUR News, February 9, 2019.

PAGE 225 *In 2016, the CDC estimated that one in two African American men:* Centers for Disease Control and Prevention, "Half of Black Gay Men and a Quarter of Latino Gay Men Projected to Be Diagnosed within Their Lifetime," press release, February 23, 2016.

PAGE 225 *More than half of all new HIV diagnoses occurred:* Linda Villarosa, "America's Hidden H.I.V. Epidemic," *New York Times,* June 6, 2017.

PAGE 226 *One explanation is that in the late 1990s, federal dollars:* Villarosa, "America's Hidden H.I.V. Epidemic."

PAGE 226 *As legal scholar Risha Foulkes has outlined:* Risha K. Foulkes, "Abstinence-Only Education and Minority Teenagers: The Importance of Race in a Question of Constitutionality," *Berkeley Journal of African-American Law and Policy* 10, no. 1 (2008): 3–51.

PAGE 226 *Zach Parolin, a researcher on poverty and social inequality:* Zach Parolin, "Welfare Money Is Paying for a Lot of Things Besides Welfare," *The Atlantic,* June 13, 2019.

PAGE 226 *The antibiotics so famously used in the US:* Tracy Kidder, *Mountains Beyond Mountains: The Quest of Dr. Paul Farmer, a Man Who Would Cure the World* (New York: Random House, 2003), 126.

PAGE 226 *Now the rate of tuberculosis in the United States is fifteen times higher:* Rebekah J. Stewart et al., "Tuberculosis—United States, 2017" *Morbidity and Mortality Weekly Report* 67, no. 11 (March 23, 2018): 317–23.

PAGE 226 *the people with tuberculosis who were born in the United States:* Stewart et al., "Tuberculosis—United States, 2017," 317–23.

PAGE 226 *In 2015, tuberculosis outranked AIDS as the leading killer:* Julie Steenhuysen, "Tuberculosis Now Rivals AIDS as Leading Cause of Death, Says WHO," *Reuters,* October 28, 2015.

PAGE 226 *two years later, New York City had its largest spike:* Marcia Frellick, "New York City Has Biggest Tuberculosis Spike in 26 Years," Medscape, March 27, 2018.

PAGE 227 *The borough of Queens—where almost half of the people are immigrants:* US Census Bureau, "QuickFacts: Queens County (Queens Borough), New York," and New York City Bureau of Tuberculosis Control, *Bureau of Tuberculosis Control Annual Summary, 2017* (Queens, NY: New York City Department of Health and Mental Hygiene, 2018).

PAGE 227 *The city's health department put the blame:* New York City Department of Health and Mental Hygiene, "Health Department Releases New Tuberculosis Data Showing 10 Percent Increase in Cases in 2017," press release, March 26, 2018.

PAGE 227 *The bacteria that cause tuberculosis have adjusted:* Helen Branswell, "Spread of Highly Drug-Resistant Tuberculosis Sparks Concerns," STAT, January 18, 2017.

PAGE 227 *New York City officials began reporting the death toll:* Jeffery C. Mays and Andy Newman, "Virus Is Twice as Deadly for Black and Latino People Than Whites in N.Y.C.," *New York Times,* April 8, 2020.

PAGE 227 *In Louisiana, 70 percent of those who died from Covid-19 were black:* Keeanga-Yamahtta Taylor, "The Black Plague," *The New Yorker,* April 16, 2020.

PAGE 227 *in Utah, where Latinx women and men constitute 14 percent:* Nate Carlisle and Sean P. Means, "With Utah Latinos Suffering COVID-19 Disproportionately, Gov. Gary Herbert Creates a Multicultural Advisory Panel," *Salt Lake Tribune,* April 23, 2020.

PAGE 227 *While a number of health officials and politicians cited:* Jossie Carreras Tartak and Hazar Khidir, "U.S. Must Avoid Building Racial Bias Into COVID-19 Emergency Guidance," NPR, April 21, 2020.

PAGE 228 *New York City's comptroller found another reason:* Mays and Newman, "Virus Is Twice as Deadly for Black and Latino People Than Whites in N.Y.C."

PAGE 229 *One morning, I clicked on a* New York Times *story:* Nelson D. Schwartz, "The Doctor Is In. Co-Pay? $40,000," *New York Times,* June 3, 2017.

PAGE 230 *If we live in a region of the country where many people:* Mark V. Pauly and José A. Pagán, "Spillovers and Vulnerability: The Case of Community Uninsurance," *Health Affairs* 26, no. 5 (September/October 2007). This is also the source for the information on studies about access to mammograms and prenatal care.

SOATÁ

PAGE 239 *She was taking fake flowers to a country:* Damian Paletta, "In Rose Beds, Money Blooms," *Washington Post,* February 10, 2018.

PAGE 240 *Colombia was taking on the kissing bug:* Andrea Marchiol et al., "Increasing Access to Comprehensive Care for Chagas Disease: Development of a Patient-Centered Model in Colombia," *Revista Panamericana de Salud Pública* 41 (December 2017).

PAGE 240 *No, Colombia did not have high rates of the disease:* World Health Organization, "Chagas Disease in Latin America: An Epidemiological Update Based on 2010 Estimates," *Weekly Epidemiological Record* 90, no. 6 (February 6, 2015) 33–43.

PAGE 240 *in 2013, it had become the first country in the world:* Marchiol et al., "Increasing Access to Comprehensive Care."

NOTES

PAGE 240 *onchocerciasis, a disease I still cannot quite comprehend:* Mark J. Taylor, Achim Hoerauf, and Moses Bockarie, "Lymphatic Filariasis and Onchocerciasis," *Lancet* 376, no. 9747 (October 2010): 1175–85.

PAGE 240 *The defeat of river blindness had apparently encouraged:* Marchiol et al., "Increasing Access to Comprehensive Care."

PAGE 240 *Along with Doctors Without Borders, they signed an agreement:* Daisy Hernández, "A New Strategy to Undermine Big Pharma's Price Gouging Actually Worked," *Slate*, September 7, 2017.

PAGE 240 *When I started packing my bags for Colombia:* Courtney Columbus, "Drug for 'Neglected' Chagas Disease Gains FDA Approval Amid Price Worries," NPR, September 10, 2017.

PAGE 241 *The company began talks to donate benznidazole:* World Health Organization, "Preventing Mother-to-Child Transmission of Chagas Disease: From Control to Elimination," November 16, 2018.

PAGE 242 *The civil war in Colombia, which had raged:* Sebastian Modak, "How Colombia, Once Consumed by Violence, Became Your Next Destination," *Condé Nast Traveler*, November 9, 2017.

PAGE 243 *The town does not have high rates of the kissing bug disease:* Marchiol et al., "Increasing Access to Comprehensive Care."

PAGE 249 *Birds are resistant to* T. cruzi: Ricardo E. Gürtler et al., "Domestic Dogs and Cats as Sources of *Trypanosoma cruzi* Infection in Rural Northwestern Argentina," *Parasitology* 134, no. 1 (January 2007): 69–82.

HER LIFE

PAGE 261 *One of the dictionaries is bilingual:* Mariano Velázquez de la Cadena et al., *New Revised Velázquez Spanish and English Dictionary* (New Jersey: New Win Publishing, 1985), 635.

NOTES

PAGE 262 *It details a dicho, or saying, that when a woman doesn't marry:* *Diccionario de la Lengua Española,* 21st ed., s.v. "Tía" (Madrid: Real Academia Española, 1992).

PAGE 262 *The saying "No hay tu tía" is thought to come from Arabic:* *Diccionario panhispánico de dudas,* 1st edition, s.v. "Tutia" (Madrid: Real Academia Española, 2005).